T0212158

Andrew Webster (*editor*)
NEW TECHNOLOGIES IN HEALTH CARE
Challenge, Change and Innovation

Andrew Webster (*editor*)
THE GLOBAL DYNAMICS OF REGENERATIVE MEDICINE
A Social Science Critique

Health, Technology and Society
Series Standing Order ISBN 978–1–403–99131–7 hardback
978–1–137–57973–7 paperback
(outside North America only)

You can receive future titles in this series as they are published by placing a stand-ing order. Please contact your bookseller or, in case of difficulty, write to us at the address below with your name and address, the title of the series and the ISBN quoted above.

Customer Services Department, Macmillan Distribution Ltd, Houndmills, Basingstoke, Hampshire RG21 6XS, England

Telecare Technologies and the Transformation of Healthcare

Nelly Oudshoorn
University of Twente, The Netherlands

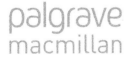

First published 2011
Published in paperback 2016 by
PALGRAVE MACMILLAN

Palgrave Macmillan in the UK is an imprint of Macmillan Publishers Limited, registered in England, company number 785998, of Houndmills, Basingstoke, Hampshire RG21 6XS.

Palgrave Macmillan in the US is a division of St Martin's Press LLC, 175 Fifth Avenue, New York, NY 10010.

Palgrave Macmillan is the global academic imprint of the above companies and has companies and representatives throughout the world.

Palgrave® and Macmillan® are registered trademarks in the United States, the United Kingdom, Europe and other countries.

ISBN 978–0–230–30020–0 hardback
ISBN 978–1–137–57972–0 paperback

This book is printed on paper suitable for recycling and made from fully managed and sustained forest sources. Logging, pulping and manufacturing processes are expected to conform to the environmental regulations of the country of origin.

A catalogue record for this book is available from the British Library.

A catalog record for this book is available from the Library of Congress.

Typeset by MPS Limited, Chennai, India.

For Rob

Contents

List of Figures and Table

Figures

Table

Acknowledgements

Although I have been fascinated by user–technology relationships for a long time, this is the first book for which I had the privilege of actually involving users in my research. Visiting patients' homes made me aware of the complexities and ambivalences people face when they are expected to use new medical technologies in times of illness. I was really impressed by patients' hospitality and openness in telling us about how telecare technologies have affected their lives or why they have rejected this new technology. Although, for privacy reasons, these heart patients remain anonymous in this book, they are the first I want to thank for sharing their experiences with academic researchers. I hope this book can contribute to making visible their pioneering work in making sense of telecare, even more so because this work is usually silenced in dominant discourses on telecare technologies.

I am also grateful to those professionally involved in the field of making telecare technologies work, particularly telecare nurses and physicians, home-care nurses, general practitioners, cardiologists and heart-failure nurses, chief executives of telecare firms, and managers of telemedical centres. In writing this book, I found their experiences and reflections to be invaluable. Without their willingness and cooperation to talk to me and allow me to observe their care practices, this book could not have been written. I am grateful, among others, to Marco Albani, Aggie Balk, Marielle de Beurs, Trix Borst, Pieter Boutkan, Pieter van der Burgh, Claudia van Dam, Cynthia Gahlert, Hanneke Glazenburg, Judith Grooters, Sandra Harthoorn, Mathilde Helm, Tony den Hollander, Leo Holwerda, Eric Jurgens, Leenders, Erwin van Leussen, Matthias Murin, Matthias Quinger, Janneke Roukema, de Ruiter, Stefan Sack, Chris van Tongeren, Anita van der Wal, Jelle van der Weijde, Dieter Wittig, and Margreet Woudenberg.

I have also benefited from the discussions and encouragement of my colleagues at the University of Twente and many colleagues and friends in the field of sociology of science and technology in Europe as well as the US. In different phases of my research, they gave inspiring and substantial comments on earlier drafts of the chapters of this book. I would like to thank Lynsey Dubbeld and Ivo Maathuis in particular for their invaluable contribution to the field work for his book. Without their careful work, creativity, and patience, it would have taken another two years before this book would have been completed. Special thanks for technical assistance are due to Hilde Meijer-Meijer, and to Gene Moore for his skilful and thorough editing of my English. I am grateful not only to people, but also to places. Places matter in writing too. Some ideas for this book were born during long walks in the dunes in Terschelling and the hills in Limburg (yes, we have hills in the Netherlands), watching migrating birds or the tide movements of the sea. Last but far from least I thank my partner, Rob Vrakking, for creating the conditions for writing this book and for sharing the pleasures of creativity. Although texts can make friends, his sculptures and drawings constitute a very special way of materializing relationships.

Some of these chapters are based on previously published material. Earlier versions of Chapters 6 and 7 have been published in *Sociology of Health & Illness*, respectively in vol. 31 (3) 2009, 390–405; and vol. 30 (2) 2008, 272–95. Parts of Chapter 2, and Chapters 7 and 8 are included in an article that will be published in *Social Studies of Science*. An earlier version of Chapter 7 has been selected as winner of the 2009 Diana Forsythe Award of the American Medical Informatics Association (AMIA). I gratefully acknowledge the permission of Hartis, Philips, and Vitaphone to use the photographs of the telecare devices investigated in this book.

Introduction
A Technogeography of Telecare

1
Who Cares?

When Mr X was diagnosed with heart failure, he felt depressed. He knew something was wrong because he was always so tired and short of breath when he did the usual things around the house. But he thought only elderly people would get this disease and he was only 57! Since the diagnosis, he feels rather useless because he also had to stop working. He even had to get rid of his pigeons because he could not feed them anymore; lifting the two-liter water can in the pigeon house made him deadly tired. But since he visited the heart-failure policlinic regularly, he felt better. The nurse showed him how to take his medicines, control his weight, and keep his diet, which helped him a lot. But last week the nurse told him that he could not visit the policlinic any longer because there were too many patients on the waiting list. Because he is doing better now, she referred him to a so-called telemedical centre. The heart-failure nurse explained that he should use a wireless scale and blood-pressure meter daily. He thought it was a kind of magic because these instruments would send his measurements automatically to the telemedical centre, where a telenurse would control them. But since this conversation he feels rather tense. Why is he no longer allowed to visit the heart-failure nurse? She was such a kind lady and she took good care of him. And what about these instruments? He did not dare to tell the nurse, but he does not feel at ease with all the new elec-tronic equipment in use nowadays. Why should he take his blood pressure himself? Why couldn't the nurse do it, as she always used to do? He wonders what he should do and phones his health insurer who runs the telemedical centre. He is told that in the near future he has to use their new health service because they will no longer reimburse his visits to the heart-failure policlinic. End of story, he thought.[1]

This scenario represents in a nutshell the changes in healthcare implied in telecare technologies. Telecare technologies enable care at a distance.[2] Patients no longer have to visit the doctor, or vice versa, because healthcare interventions are mediated by information and communication technologies (ICTs). In the past decade, the healthcare sector in modern societies has witnessed the testing and introduction of an increasing number of telecare applications aimed at monitoring and diagnosing a variety of chronic diseases, including diabetes, respiratory insufficiency, and heart diseases.[3] The introduction of these new technological devices has major consequences for healthcare. The most drastic change involves a transformation in the order of care. Who cares in the scenario of telecare technologies described above? Obviously, acts of care are no longer restricted to doctors and nurses: patients are expected to play an active role as well. Telecare technologies imply that patients perform tasks previously delegated to healthcare professionals. The telecare devices for heart patients investigated in this book require that patients conduct their own electrocardiograms (ECGs), take their own blood pressure, or measure their weight themselves. The use of telecare devices disciplines patients to inspect their own bodies regularly and to integrate these activities into their daily routines at home. The scenario also illustrates that care is delegated not only to patients but also to a new category of healthcare professionals: telenurses. They are expected to act as intermediaries between patients, telecare devices, and healthcare professionals – in this case heart-failure nurses and cardiologists. Although newspaper headlines such as 'Computer replaces cardiologist' try to make us believe that telecare technologies do not require any human intervention current telecare technologies depend on specially trained nurses (Anonymous, 2003). The introduction of this new technology involves a proliferation of the work required to read and interpret more and more diagnostic and monitoring data. Healthcare is thus no longer solely in the hands of traditional healthcare professionals but becomes distributed among a variety of different actors, including patients and telenurses.

The scenario of telecare technology involves not only multiple actors; it also indicates how care can be dispersed over different locations. As a result of the introduction of telecare technologies, healthcare is no longer restricted to the hospital or a general practitioner's consulting room but also includes patients' homes and telecare centres. These new sites of care are populated not only by people but also by a variety of technical devices, including computers, electronic triage systems, telemonitoring systems, and various electronic devices for measuring key diagnostic markers. Telecare technologies thus imply multiple sites, multiple actors, and multiple technological objects. Consequently, the seemingly straightforward question of 'who cares?' does not have a simple answer. Telecare technologies require complex interactions and create multiple interdependencies between people and things which transform healthcare as we used to know it. This book aims to trace these changes by describing how telecare technologies redefine the order of care, change the identity of healthcare professionals and patients, and transform care itself.

Multiple sites of care: From home to hospital and back home again?

One of the changes implied in telecare technologies is that they extend the reach of healthcare to locations outside the hospital and the physician's consulting room. One of these sites is the patient's home. This shift towards the home is one of the selling features of the new technology, as is exemplified by the slogan 'Bringing it all back home' used by one of the leading international electronic firms involved in the development and introduction of telecare technologies (Philips flyer, 2005). From a historical perspective, the transfer of healthcare from hospital to home is very intriguing. Prior to the 1800s, healthcare was 'bedside medicine', where doctors visited patients at home to diagnose and treat diseases. From the 1840s patient care gradually moved to hospitals (Nettleton, 2004). It is thus not the first time that the patient's home is seen as an important location for healthcare. In the shifts of healthcare from home to hospital and, vice versa, technologies have played a major role. Historians of medicine have characterized the 1850s–1890s as the period during which medical technologies and laboratory tests came to dominate healthcare. Instruments initially used for scientific research, adapted for medical use by a growing number of new industries and businesses that specialized in medical techniques, gradually penetrated healthcare. Doctors increasingly relied on medical instruments which, together with chemical laboratory tests of urine and blood, came more and more to replace physical examinations in diagnosing diseases. In addition to the stethoscope, the thermometer, and the microscope, doctors used electro-physiological diagnostic instruments, electrotherapy, and surgical instruments. The introduction of these new diagnostic and therapeutic instruments and the emergence of laboratories led to a drastic reorganization of healthcare, including the rise of the modern hospital, which became a key site of healthcare (Houwaart, 2001).

The current move of healthcare from hospitals to patients' homes is not only facilitated by telecare technologies but is also related to other technologies. Health reforms in industrialized countries aimed at reducing the length of hospital stays in order to decrease healthcare spending have resulted in an increased use of specialized medical instruments at home (Lehoux et al., 2004; Arras et al., 1995). These medical instruments include devices for the treating acute infectious diseases, such as antibiotic intravenous therapy, which are used for a short period. There are also instruments for chronic conditions or terminal diseases, which are used for longer periods, such as instruments for terminal renal failure and oxygen therapy (Lehoux et al., 2004, p. 618). Medical sociologists have described how 'high-tech home-care' involves much more than just transferring a particular medical technology from hospital to home. It requires the delegation and redistribution of skills, knowledge, and devices to places considered private and safe, spaces in which medical instruments are often perceived as necessary but nevertheless threatening intruders (Angus et al., 2005; Lehoux et al., 2004; Cartier, 2003; Heaton et al. 2005). In addition to high-tech home-care technologies, a growing number of self-care technologies have become available for patients who suffer from less severe chronic diseases, such as the metered-dose inhaler for asthma patients (Willems, 1995; Prout, 1996).

Like home-care and self-care technologies, telecare technologies also position the home as the key site for technology-mediated healthcare. Advocates of the new technology promise that the clinic will be taken out of its built walls and delivered to the doorsteps of its spatially distributed clientele. As Brown and Webster have described, this view of the clinic's being transferred to the patient's home has been a long-held ambition and dream of medical technologists (Brown and Webster, 2004, p. 86). Telecare technologies not only follow the path of homecare and self-care technologies, but are also shaped by ICT-based technologies used in contemporary clinics, such as diagnostic imaging and monitoring technologies. The major difference is that telecare technologies take the imaging and surveillance technologies outside the hospital and bring them into the patient's home. Equally importantly, medical inspection of bodies is no longer restricted to medical experts but is partly delegated to patients. In the process, telecare technologies make patients active in 'gazing into their own bodies' (Langstrup Nielsen, 2003, p. 20). This is an important departure from medical practices at home prior to the nineteenth century. Although the home is a key site for healthcare in both periods, the use of medical technologies is no longer restricted to medical experts – since the 1990s patients have been expected to use medical instruments themselves.

History, therefore, is not repeating itself. Compared to the nineteenth century, there is not only a shift in agency from doctors to patients; there is also an important difference in the way the home is positioned in the infrastructure of healthcare. Although the inspection of bodies takes place at home, the results of these acts of care are not only included in the notebook of the doctor, as happened in the nineteenth and far into the twentieth century, but are distributed over a large network of different actors and locations, thus extending the spatial (and temporal) boundaries of healthcare. ECGs, graphs of blood pressure and weight measures, images of skin, and other representations of the body may be registered at home, but the interpretation of these data takes place elsewhere. ICT-based healthcare technologies transfer data to specialist departments and laboratories in hospitals and the newly established telemedical centres, where healthcare professionals analyse and control data. The outcome of the inspection of bodies is thus not only accessible to doctors but is dispersed over many actors, which creates a radical availability of the body not only for clinical but also for research and health insurance purposes (Brown and Webster, 2004). Compared to previous centuries, the home is no longer an isolated, independent site of healthcare but is practically and materially integrated by imaging and digital technologies with acts of care at hospitals, general practitioners' rooms, laboratories, and telemedical centres. The expression 'bringing it all back home' is thus inadequate to capture the changes in healthcare implied in telecare technologies. In a similar vein, the phrase 'move from hospital to home' is not appropriate because it suggests that healthcare is taken away from one site to be performed elsewhere. Equally problematically, this rhetoric suggests that telecare devices can be applied only at home. However, the use of telecare technologies is not restricted to the home; some telecare devices can be used when patients are on the move, or are designed explicitly to increase the mobility of patients. Telecare technologies will therefore be used not only at home but carried around to many other places, including work spaces, shopping malls, holiday cottages, or the homes of family and friends. Although we should therefore be careful in describing the changes in healthcare implied in telecare technologies as moving care from hospital to home, the home is nevertheless becoming more prominent in healthcare.

Another important site for telecare technologies is the telemedical centre. Although the evaluation and processing of measurements collected by patients can take place in hospitals or general practitioners' rooms, the data are often transferred to telemedical centres. As such, the telemedical centre is not a complete novelty in healthcare but can be considered as an extension of health services delivered by using the telephone. Telephone-based health services, usually run by nurses, have existed since the 1970s. The introduction of computer-supported clinical assessment systems further facilitated the emergence of health services based on non-face-to-face interactions between healthcare providers and patients. Since the early 1990s, many European countries, the US, and Canada have introduced telephone-based health services, usually referred to as 'medical call centres'.[4] In the UK, for example, the National Health Service (NHS) introduced NHS Direct, a nurse-based, 24-hour health-advice line initiated by the NHS. People who are worried about their health can phone these centres to discuss health problems and receive advice about the most appropriate care (Hanlon et al., 2005. Medical call centres can be located at SOS emergency organizations or regular healthcare organizations (Wahlberg et al., 2003, p. 38). Telemedical centres can be considered a further extension of the services provided by medical call centres, but innovators in telemedicine usually resist this comparison because of the negative responses to call centres.[5] Consequently, actors who operate telemedical centres carefully avoid any association with medical call centres by referring to their organizations as medical service centres or telemedical centres rather than medical call centres. Of course, this use of another term is not only a rhetorical or political strategy. Telemedical centres differ from medical call centres because they are based on different technologies and deliver other services. Whereas medical call centres are based on telephones, computers, and clinical assessment software programs, and only give health advice, telemedical centres are usually based on a combination of old media technologies (telephone and TV), new media technologies (internet, webcams), and telemedical devices (electronic weight scales, blood pressure meters, and ECG devices) and provide both diagnostic and monitoring care services.

We can conclude, therefore, that the home and telemedical centres are important sites at which healthcare mediated by telecare technologies takes place.

Multiple actors: Who controls the clinical gaze?

Telecare devices not only distribute care over different sites, they also depend on multiple actors. Although advocates of the new technology try to convince us that telecare technologies reduce human labour because work is partly delegated to technological devices (e.g. Bauer and Ringel, 1999; Wootton, 2000), this representation of telemedicine and telecare technologies is problematic because it makes invisible all the work involved in operating these new technologies. As sociologists of science, technology and medicine have described, the introduction of new technologies often leads to a redistribution rather than a reduction of work. As early as 1981, Illich suggested that 'work does not disappear with technological aid. Rather it is displaced – sometimes onto the machine, as often onto workers' (Illich, 1981). The introduction of new technologies in healthcare can thus be expected to play an important role in delegating and redistributing tasks among healthcare professionals, between healthcare professionals and patients, and between people and technological devices. Recent studies of telemedical technologies have shown how the delegation of work is indeed a major characteristic of this new technology. Maggie Mort et al. (2003) have described how the introduction of telemedical devices in the dermatological clinic leads to a redistribution of interactional work with patients from dermatologists to nurses. In a similar vein, Lisa Cartwright has suggested that in telemediated healthcare nurses and physicians' assistants are key actors who have to perform many tasks in the absence of physicians (Cartwright, 2000). The work involved in providing healthcare at a distance is delegated not only to nurses or physicians' assistants, but also to healthcare professionals outside the traditional healthcare infrastructure of clinics and physicians' consultation rooms, namely the new category of telecare worker.

One major consequence of the introduction of telecare technologies is that more actors become involved in healthcare. The use of the telecare technologies investigated in this book involves cardiologists, heart-failure nurses, general practitioners, home-care nurses, telenurses, telephysicians, health-insurance companies, telemedical firms, and, last but not least, patients. Diagnostic and monitoring work thus becomes dispersed over an extensive network of actors, including technical devices that connect previously separated locations such as the consulting rooms of general practitioners and clinicians, the offices of home-care nurses and heart-failure nurses, polyclinics and the emergency departments of hospitals, telemedical centres, and patients' homes. This distributed character of healthcare challenges the traditional role of the carer Who should be considered as the primary carer when care is dispersed over different groups of actors, including patients and the new category of telecare professionals? Or to rephrase this in Foucauldian terms: Who controls the clinical gaze when healthcare is distributed over different actors and locations? Based on the insights of research on user–technology relations, we might expect that the heterogeneous users of telecare technologies will not necessarily share the same views of the new technology.[6] Although all users can be considered as active participants in implementing and using telecare technologies, they do not occupy the same position in the emerging landscape of care. Equally importantly, the technological devices will delegate certain actions to one group of users, while denying these actions to others. There is also an important difference in terms of whose bodies are affected by the new technology. Whereas healthcare professionals, health insurers, and telemedical firms relate to the new technology in the context of work only, the patients' use of telecare devices includes a direct intervention in their own bodies and homes.

In this respect it is important to consider whether patients can be considered as users. As Pascale Lehoux et al. (2004) have suggested for high-tech home-care technologies, the use of a technology aimed at facilitating tasks in a work environment may be different from the use of medical devices that support the maintenance of the body for chronic, sometimes life-threatening diseases at home. The actions of patients involved in monitoring and producing diagnosis can thus not be considered merely in terms of performing tasks, particularly if this implies the adoption of a purely functional perspective (Lehoux et al., 2004, p. 621). Telecare technologies do much more than act as functional tools to monitor data; they transform the relationship between patients and their bodies. This is because patients are expected to become more active and responsible as participants in the diagnosis and monitoring of their disorders.

To be sure, telecare technologies should not be considered a novelty because they delegate the use of medical devices to patients. Patients are already familiar with the use of various medical instruments, including home-care and self-care technologies. There is, however, an important difference between telecare technologies and devices such as the inhaler for asthma or the familiar thermometer. Whereas using a thermometer or an asthma inhaler can be considered as isolated individual acts that patients can perform wherever and whenever they prefer, the use of telecare devices is materially and morally integrated into a network of care that guides and restricts the actions of patients. Social studies of technology suggest that the same instruments can have a different identity and meaning when integrated into different practices (Law, 1999; Prout, 1996; Pols, 2008). Consequently, the use of a blood-pressure meter in a telecare setting is different from using a blood-pressure meter at home during a period of flu or for monitoring physical exercises during sport. Telecare technologies aim to discipline patients to inspect their bodies regularly by inscribing the required actions in technological devices that are subsequently controlled by healthcare professionals and technical devices.

Telecare technologies not only disturb the order of care because they delegate acts of care previously performed by doctors to patients; they also intervene in relationships among healthcare professionals. Because of the diversity of the healthcare professionals involved in telecare technologies, the implementation of these new technologies is likely to become a site of struggle about who controls the clinical gaze. Do healthcare professionals accept the tasks and responsibilities delegated to them and others, particularly the newcomers? For traditional healthcare professionals,[7] telecare technologies imply that some of the care they used to provide to patients is now delegated to telecare professionals and telemedical centres. Telecare technologies thus challenge the professional autonomy and authority of traditional healthcare providers. Moreover, whereas the diagnosis and monitoring of heart patients used to be the domain of cardiologists, general practitioners, and specialized nurses, this care is partly delegated to the new profession of telecare workers. Based on the literature of the sociology of medical professions, we might expect traditional healthcare providers to try to maintain their authority over their qualifications (Abbott, 1988). The new technology disrupts the order of care because it intervenes in long-established traditions and vested interests in healthcare. It thus seems likely that the introduction of telecare technologies may result in inter-disciplinary contests between traditional healthcare professionals and the newcomers in the field of care for heart patients. Telecare workers are not entering an empty, uncontested space. They are likely to meet resistance to their work and to their becoming accepted as new actors in healthcare. Moreover, they are not the only category of healthcare workers recently introduced into healthcare. Since the 1980s there has been an increased reliance on intermediary

actors in healthcare, including nurse practitioners and other specialized nurses such as heart-failure nurses. Telecare technologies followed
this trend by introducing telenurses and telephysicians. A major difference between nurse practitioners and heart-failure nurses, however,
is that telecare workers are not integrated into existing healthcare
organizations such as general practitioners' rooms or polyclinics, but
that they work in the newly established infrastructure of telemedical
centres.

Telemedical centres are a novelty not only because of the kind of
work performed in these places, but also because they are established,
owned, and run by commercial players in healthcare, i.e., health insurers and the telemedical industry. The order of care is thus challenged
also because actors from the private sector are intervening in spaces
that used to belong to the public sector, at least in Europe.[8] Although
health insurance companies and medical industries have always played
a major role in healthcare, the introduction of telecare technologies
implies an important new role for these actors: instead of producing
technical devices or reimbursing the costs of healthcare, telemedical
companies, and health insurers are adopting the role of owners and
managers of healthcare organizations. By establishing and operating
telemedical centres, these actors become repositioned in the landscape
of care and assume a hybrid identity of respectively producers-caregivers
and insurers-caregivers. This new configuration drastically challenges
the established conventions and boundaries between the public and
the private sectors. Again, it seems likely that the established medical
professions will not readily accept these changes. Telecare technologies
thus challenge the order of care because they create novel interdependencies between old and new actors.

In this reordering of care, gender is also implicated. As feminist
scholars have demonstrated, the healthcare sector shows a gendered
segregation of labour in which men still dominate the higher management positions and, to a lesser extent, the clinical professionals,
whereas women dominate the nursing and medical assistant professions (Armstrong et al., 2007, 2009). We may therefore wonder whether
and how the new category of telecare workers challenges or reinforces
this gendered hierarchy in healthcare. Equally importantly, we may
wonder how the move in healthcare from the clinic to the home shapes
gender divisions of care work in households. Feminist studies in the
sociology and geography of health have shown that informal care work
has been constructed as a female activity and responsibility. In many
cultures, women not only take responsibility for their own health but

also shoulder the major responsibility for taking care of the health of their male partners, children, and usually other family members (Doyal, 2001; Annandale and Kuhlman, 2010; Milligan, 2001, 2009). This raises the important question of whether and how telecare technologies contribute to shaping gendered patterns of care work at home.[9]

The political economy of telecare: Chronic diseases and neo-liberalization of healthcare

Who cares about telecare technologies? Whose interests are at stake? The involvement of healthcare insurers and the medical industry, not only as insurers and producers but also as actors who operate telemedical centres, suggests a specific political economy of care in which the development and introduction of telecare technologies takes place. Why should health insurance and medical companies be interested in running healthcare organizations? One key explanation for these hybrid functions concerns the rising costs and reduced profits of healthcare. Over the past three decades, controlling and decreasing healthcare spending has been a major concern for healthcare insurers, governmental agencies, and managers of healthcare organizations in Western industrialized countries; they have been at pains to reduce fears that the provision of healthcare is no longer affordable. This is not the place to discuss the economics of healthcare in detail, but it is important to note how telecare technologies are related to these problems. Telecare devices are developed and introduced at the intersection of three related discourses that are mobilized as resources to articulate the importance and identity of the new technology: the discourse on an increase in chronic diseases due to an ageing population; the discourse on the modernization and rationalization of healthcare work; and the discourse on the neo-liberalization of healthcare.

The first discourse emphasizes that financing healthcare will become increasingly difficult because of demographic changes. As the population grows older, national health authorities and international public health organizations such as the World Health Organization (WHO) expect a rise in chronic diseases, resulting in a growing demand for care (European Commission, 2007).In Europe, important policy and funding agencies such as the European Commission (EC) support the development of telemedical technologies and refer to them as 'innovative technologies for chronic disease management. Or, as the director of the EC's Information Society and New Media articulated this concern at a conference organized in Brussels in December 2007 to launch the EC's initiative to develop a future action plan for telemedicine: 'Everyone in Europe is getting older and chronic diseases are on the rise. A telemedical initiative could offer a constructive way of dealing with these growing challenges' (European Commission, 2007, p. 8). In his address to the conference, the director warned the EU Member States that if they did not address these problems, Europe would no longer be able to afford healthcare within the available budgets. The basic message of this discourse is that healthcare will no longer be affordable because of the lack of available resources, not only in terms of budgets abut also because of a scarcity of healthcare professionals. Telecare technologies are then positioned as important means of bridging the gap between the growing demand for care for chronic diseases due to an ageing population and the expected scarcity of human and financial resources. Telecare technologies are expected to bridge this gap by delegating care work to telecare devices and by moving the monitoring of the health of chronic patients to the patients' homes, which may prevent expensive hospitalization.

The second discourse concerns the modernization and rationalization of healthcare work. In this discourse, telecare technologies, and other ICTs, are positioned as tools to make healthcare more efficient by rationalizing work. The introduction of ICTs in healthcare will save money because they will standardize health services and make them more routine (Timmermans and Berg, 2003). ICTs introduced to support communication and information exchange among healthcare professionals and between healthcare providers and patients are expected to improve the workflow and reduce the workload of doctors and nurses. A major argument in this discourse is that healthcare can become more cost-effective by delegating work from expensive medical experts to less expensive, specialized nurses, and moving healthcare from the hospital to primary care. Computer-supported decision programs, for example, are expected to shift routine work away from clinicians to specialized nurses affiliated to medical call centres (May et al., 2005, p. 1490). Telecare devices are expected to reduce healthcare spending because they move the care provided to hospital outpatients into primary care and to the new category of telecare workers.

Telecare and other ICT-based healthcare services are considered not only as tools to make healthcare more cost-effective by delegating work to technical devices and redistributing work among professionals; they are also expected to reduce costs by delegating expensive care to the patients themselves (Timmermans and Berg, 2003).

This shift to patients is related to the third discourse mobilized by advocates of telecare technologies: a neoliberalization of healthcare.

In the past two decades, the healthcare sector in Western industrialized countries has adopted neoliberal politics in which health is considered to be the personal responsibility of citizens. Individuals are expected to take responsibility for their own health, to tackle chronic diseases and reduce healthcare spending, a message conveyed by leading public-sector agencies such as the WHO (Nettleton, 2006, p. 238). In this discourse, healthcare provision is redefined as a market driven by individual demands and the ability of citizens to pay for healthcare services (Lehoux, 2006, p. xxv). As a consequence, all aspects of healthcare are described in terms of commodity exchange; healthcare provision is presented as healthcare service, and patients are transformed into consumers or clients (Brown and Webster, 2004). Medical sociologists have described these changes as the emergence of a 'consumerist' type of healthcare in which medicine is framed as a 'commodity, chosen by individuals, usually in free markets' (Pickstone, 2000, p. 3).[10] This neoliberalization of healthcare introduces new ways in which healthcare technologies, including telecare technologies, are produced and used. The individualization of healthcare, in which health is defined as a personal responsibility or lifestyle choice, implies that healthcare technologies become subject to and are shaped by the economic interests of the medical industry and health insurance companies rather than by national governmental politics or state funding. Consequently, the relationship between healthcare providers and users of healthcare technologies is redefined as a contractual relationship rather than a public service. Healthcare technologies, like other healthcare provisions, are turned into consumer services rather than doctor-prescribed treatments (Brown and Webster, 2004, p. 51, 84).

Although neoliberalization politics in healthcare is embraced by many countries with advanced economies, including the US, Canada, and Western Europe, there are important national differences. Whereas consumerist and fee-based payments for healthcare are a major characteristic of healthcare in the US, neoliberal tendencies have emerged more recently in European countries, including the UK, Germany, and the Netherlands. The political culture in these European countries is, however, quite different from that in the US in accepting a more central role for the national state in providing healthcare (Brown and Webster, 2004; Bijker, 2007).[11] Despite these differences, telecare technologies are promoted as important instruments for realizing a market approach to healthcare in Europe as well as the US. Illustrative of this move towards the neo-liberalization of healthcare in Europe is the European Commission's description of the development and implementation of telemedical technologies, which they stimulate and partly finance, as making important contributions to the EU economy (European Commission, 2008, p. 689). In Germany and the Netherlands, some of the telecare devices for heart patients investigated in this book are explicitly promoted to individual consumers. The German telemedical company Vitaphone has introduced a telecare device that individuals can buy via the firm's website. In the Netherlands, with its long tradition of doctor-prescribed medical treatments, one health insurance company with a telemedical centre promotes its telecare services as follows:

> The developments relating to remote healthcare fit in well with the changes in the health system initiated by the Dutch government. The developments are aimed at promoting the operation of market forces and liberalization of the health market. The increased influence of market forces and liberalization are key success factors for the launch of this new model of healthcare delivery.
>
> (Montfoort and Helm, 2006, p. 35)

In the emerging political economy of telecare, the new technology is thus framed as an instrument to support the liberalization of healthcare, to modernize and rationalize healthcare work, and to attune healthcare resources to the growing demand for healthcare among an ageing population. Increasing the efficiency and reducing the costs of healthcare are important and relevant concerns. Changes in healthcare may be required to reduce the gap between the growing demand for care and shrinking resources, in terms of both financial and human capital. The problem, however, is that the representation of telecare technologies as serving narrow economic interests reflects and reinforces a reductionist view of healthcare that hides other changes in healthcare implicated in telecare technologies. What actually happens when healthcare becomes distributed over different places and actors, including technical devices? What are the consequences for healthcare when care partly shifts from physical to virtual encounters between healthcare providers and patients? These are urgent questions that tend to be neglected when telecare technologies are represented only as efficient economic tools.

Discourses on the political economy of telecare not only reflect a specific approach to healthcare; they also imply a specific view of technology that presents an obstacle to understanding how new technologies affect healthcare. The next chapter therefore criticizes this view and introduces an alternative conceptualization of the complex relationship between technology and transformations in healthcare. Moreover, the chapter describes the research questions and method, and also the organization of this book.

2
Theorizing Technology and the Transformation of Healthcare

Telecare devices as problem solvers?

The discourses on telecare described in the previous chapter reflect not only a reductionist view of healthcare; they also rely on a rather restricted view of technology. Actors with vested interests in the promotion of telecare technologies consider these innovations as problem solvers: telecare devices are expected to make healthcare more efficient and affordable. These discourses thus reinforce an instrumental view of technology: technologies are considered as tools that make it possible to realize a specific aim. The history of technology, however, shows many examples of technologies that don't do what innovators want them to do. Over the past two decades, social studies of user–technology relationships have described the discrepancies between how technologies were initially meant to be used and how users modified technical devices to meet their own goals (Oudshoorn and Pinch, 2003, 2007). The instrumental view of technology, which assumes a direct, causal relationship between aim and effects, has also been criticized because it fails to recognize that technologies transform problems rather than solve them. For example, the introduction of telecare technologies designed to reduce costs by delegating healthcare work partly to patients, telecare workers, and technological devices, may actually increase rather than decrease healthcare spending because the use of telecare technologies may increase the number of diagnoses that require medical treatment. Also, the availability of telecare technologies may lead to an increase in the use of these devices in cases where there is no strict medical need (Willems, 2006). Although technologies may contribute to the promises of its producers, they may also do other things. Telecare technologies not only affect the political economy of healthcare; they also intervene

17

in the order of care by distributing care over multiple places and actors and creating networks between people and things. However, these networks do not operate by themselves: the technology works only when all the actors and technical devices perform the actions delegated to them. Telecare technologies cannot thus be considered as mere instrumental tools for the more efficient delivery of healthcare. On the contrary, they should be considered as active agents that participate in changing the order of healthcare and what care is all about. This kind of agency of technology is not taken into account in the instrumental view of technology.

The approach that inspired me, and which is developed further in this book, suggests an alternative conceptualization of the relationship between technologies and change. Instead of the instrumental view, I adopt a material–semiotic approach[1] in order to understand how technologies act as socio-cultural agents. In this approach, technologies are considered not as tools that solve problems, but as actants that transform them by redefining the nature of the problem and the identities of the people and objects considered relevant to solving the problem. This transformative quality of technology is not an inherent capacity of technical devices but the result of the socio-cultural dynamics of the networks in which technologies are supposed to act (Callon, 1985; Latour, 1989, 2005). Technologies work only when they are embedded in heterogeneous networks in which people, organizations, knowledge, skills, and technological devices interact to produce a specific practice of work, or, in the case of telecare technology, a practice of care (Latour, 1988, 1989, 2005; Mol, 2002, Mol et al., 2010; Law, 1999, 2008). Following this perspective, technologies can no longer be considered as isolated instruments that determine economic or socio-cultural change; rather they emerge in heterogeneous networks in which humans and objects interact to produce specific socio-technical practices (Latour, 1990, 2005). This approach enables me to understand how technologies contribute to reconfiguring the actions and interdependencies between people and technological devices involved in telecare technologies. From a material–semiotic perspective, the delegation and redistribution of agency among people and objects emerge as key features in understanding how technologies contribute to socio-cultural change.

In order to capture how technologies participate in delegating and (re)distributing actions, competencies, and responsibilities among people and between people and objects, Madeleine Akrich has introduced the concept of 'script'. Comparing technologies to film, Akrich suggests that 'like a film script, technical objects define a framework of action together with the actors and the space in which they are supposed to act' (Akrich, 1992, p. 208). To explain how scripts of technological objects emerge, she draws our attention to the design of technologies. In the design phase, engineers, and other actors, construct images of users and use and objectify these representations in technological choices. The inscription of representations of users and use in artefacts results in technologies that contain a script: they attribute and delegate specific competencies, actions, and responsibilities to users and technological devices (Akrich, 1992, p. 208). This semiotics of technological objects provides a useful heuristic to understand how telecare technologies challenge the existing order and create a new order of care. Adopting this approach, I conceptualize telecare technologies as active participants in shifting agency and responsibilities among doctors, nurses, patients, and technical devices, creating new 'geographies of responsibilities' (Akrich, 1992, p. 207). Changes in the order of 'who cares' can thus be understood in terms of challenges to, and transformations of, existing geographies of responsibilities in healthcare. The core of the research presented in this book traces these changing geographies by analysing the ways in which technical objects modify existing and create novel connections and interdependencies between the people and the technological objects involved in providing healthcare.

A second relevant feature of the material–semiotic approach to technology is that technical devices and people don't have intrinsic, preordained qualities that are defined once and for all. In socio-technical networks, neither human actors nor technological objects are stable. The elements that constitute these networks acquire their characteristics or identities only as part of these networks. Socio-technical networks order, arrange, and create linkages between actors and identities, ascribing and distributing properties and qualities to people and objects. In this view of technology, there are no causal, linear, constitutive relationships between humans and objects; they define each other mutually rather than causing one another (Callon, 1985; Latour, 1987, 2005; Law, 1999, 2008). People and technological objects interact continuously according to the actions and competencies delegated to them, which may be contested but nevertheless shape who they are and what they do. Without telecare technologies, telenurses and remote healthcare do not exist, and vice versa: without patients acting as inspectors of their bodies, telecare technologies do not exist.

Technologies thus change not only the relationships between people and technological objects by reconfiguring their actions and interdependencies; they also (re)define their identities in terms of what care is all about. Like other healthcare technologies, telecare technologies deeply transform how humans work, live, and cope with diseases.[2] As sociologists of technology and medicine have described, the use of health technologies modifies the collective and individual identities of patients. Genetic technologies, for example, are changing definitions of kinship and inheritance. Reproductive technologies are drastically transforming long-standing practices and definitions of motherhood and what counts as the beginning of life (Lehoux, 2006; Brown and Webster, 2004; Franklin and Ragone, 1998). Unravelling how telecare technologies participate as socio-cultural agents in the construction of new healthcare configurations, including professional identities, patient identities, and new forms of care, increases our understanding of how new health technologies transform the world we live in. This book therefore aims to explore what kind of patients, doctors, nurses, technological objects, and forms of care are constituted in the emerging socio-technical networks of telecare technologies.

The conceptualization of technologies as socio-cultural agents rather than problem solvers is not only of theoretical relevance. Telecare technologies also have an explicit political agenda: they aim to increase the efficiency of healthcare and make care more affordable. These goals can be realized only when current healthcare practices are (partly) replaced by telecare technologies. This replacement agenda is problematic because it assumes that telecare technologies act only as mediators of human interaction and merely facilitate healthcare delivery. As Mort et al. (2004) have described, advocates of telemedical technologies, including policymakers, perceive telemedicine and telecare to be about technology rather than about medicine; they consider the new technology merely in terms of tools that facilitate the delivery of healthcare. This rhetoric of delivery thus reinforces the image of technology as isolated instruments that can simply be inserted and diffused in healthcare without changing what care is all about. In this book I argue that telecare cannot be considered as a replication of existing healthcare. Instead I show how telecare technologies participate in constituting different kinds of care, healthcare professionals, and patients.

Technogeography of care

This study of telecare technologies not only builds on insights developed in science and technology studies (STS) but is also inspired by human geography. This field of expertise recognizes the importance of place in defining human relationships.[3] Human geographers understand place as a site of social relations: 'places are not just physical but also involve situated human intention with them' (Andrews, 2003). Like STS, human geography goes beyond deterministic views by emphasizing that people and places are mutually constitutive (McKeever, 2001, p. 4). Places act as sites of social relations, and human relationships have spatial aspects: 'our proximity to or distance from others and from places have meaning for us' (Malone, 2003, p. 2317). The view that places matter has also been adopted and further elaborated on by scholars in the field of health geography to emphasize 'the emplaced nature' of healthcare (Milligan, 2009, p. 6; 2001; Andrews, 2002, 2003; Poland et al., 2005).[4] According to Christine Milligan, healthcare should be understood within a 'relational framework' in which the practices of care-givers and care-recipients are investigated in relation to the places in which care takes place (Milligan et al., 2007, p. 135). This scholarship has been very important in drawing attention to contemporary changes in the institutional spaces in healthcare, particularly the shift to community-based care and the redistribution of care from the state and formal care-givers to informal care-givers such as voluntary organizations and the family, due to welfare state reforms in advanced industrialized countries in the past two decades. This shifting landscape of care, often referred to as 'extitutionalization', requires a rethinking of the distinctions between formal and informal care practices that take place in institutional spaces such as the hospital, the community, and the home (Milligan, 2009, p. 23; Mort, Finch and May, 2009, p. 11). As Pascale Lehoux and colleagues have argued, the very places where care takes place shape how informal and formal caregivers 'define their technical, moral, and professional duties, and how they behave' (Lehoux et al., 2004, p. 644).

Although this scholarship thus provides important insights into the relationships between people, place and care, the role of technology in the changing landscape of healthcare has been neglected for a long time. In the agenda-setting paper *How place matters*, Poland and colleagues conclude that the ways in which technologies affect place is often not recognized in social studies of healthcare (Poland et al., 2005). Reflecting on the different approaches to technology and health, particularly phenomenological perspectives on human–technology relations, the authors emphasize the importance of place in understanding how technologies mediate or interfere with the experiences of patients and healthcare professionals, thus enabling or constraining 'empowerment, resistance, and the extension of power and social control' (Poland et al., 2005, p. 176). One of the first empirical studies to investigate the relationships between place, care and technology is the study of Lisa Cartwright on telemedicine in the US and Canada, in which she argued that telemedical technologies introduce a 'new geography of local and global health promotion management' (Cartwright, 2000, p. 348). Cartwright showed how telemedicine constitutes new configurations of community identity and populations, including new definitions of remote peoples. Whereas Cartwright refers to 'geography of care' to describe how telemedicine affects populations, more recent studies employ a geographical approach to study the local telecare practices and lived experiences of care-givers and care-recipients. Maggie Mort, Celia Roberts, Christine Milligan, and Daniel Lopez, for example, focused on telecare and domestic technologies developed for frail, elderly people in order to understand how these new care technologies contribute to reallocating care to the domestic home, introducing new responsibilities and new actors, and creating new meanings of 'ageing in place' (Mort et al., 2009; Milligan, 2009; Roberts and Mort, 2009; Mort et al., 2008; Milligan et al., 2010; Lopez, 2010). These studies described how technologically advanced surveillance systems, such as motion and fall detectors introduced to enable frail elderly people to remain in their homes for longer and to reduce the potential risks of living independently at home, create and reconfigure 'spaces of care', including care homes and private homes. This scholarship shows how these technologies contribute to changing the landscape of care by rearranging the traditional boundaries between institutional and non-institutional settings, in which homes become institutionalized, whereas traditional care institutions become more home-like (Schillmeijer and Domenech, 2010, pp. 2, 6). Most importantly, this scholarship illustrates the relevance of adopting a geographical approach by showing how these surveillance technologies contribute to a profound change in how elderly people sense and experience their homes (Milligan et al., 2010; Schillmeijer and Domenech, 2010, p. 5). Whereas these scholars have focused on telecare technologies for elderly people, the research presented in this book aims to contribute to this important, emerging field of study by addressing telecare technologies for patients. Telecare technologies invade not only the homes of the elderly but also the homes of (chronic) patients, which, taken together, are indicative of the pervasive character of these new care technologies in industrialized societies.

Adopting a focus on place is thus important to understanding how technologies participate in changing the landscape of healthcare. This book therefore aims to build bridges between STS and human geography by including place as an important element in shaping user–technology relations. Scripts of technology may be important in pre-structuring human actions, but, adopting the insights of human geographers, we should be aware that places are also important. Places are not only important because assumptions about the contexts of use are inscribed in technologies, as Akrich has argued.[5] They also matter because places may shape how technological devices are used, or not, and (de)stabilize the specific identities of technologies. Equally importantly, technologies, in turn, may participate in redefining the meaning and practices of the spaces in which they are used and, as I will show, introduce new spaces in which people and objects interact. The view that places matter thus provides an important point of departure for investigating how reciprocal relationships between places and technologies enable or constrain the creation of specific professional and patient identities and forms of care.

A focus on places is particularly relevant to understanding how telecare technologies reorder and redefine healthcare. Although other medical technologies also affect the spatial dimensions of healthcare, telecare technologies do this in a very specific way. These technologies redefine the spatial dimensions of healthcare by (re)distributing healthcare over multiple locations and actors. Although the dispersal of care can also be observed in current healthcare practices, telecare technologies introduce a situation in which care is distributed over different locations and actors but is simultaneously connected by ICTs. Telecare technologies imply a transformation of healthcare because they create networks in a literal, material sense: actors and places are connected by various technologies that operate via copper wires, glass fibres, and satellites. Consequently, telecare technologies introduce very explicit and forceful scripts for collaboration and interdependencies. The most crucial way in which telecare technologies affect the spatial dimensions of healthcare is that acts of care such as diagnosis and monitoring take place when healthcare providers and patients are not in the same place. Compared to other technology-mediated healthcare practices, geographical distance is integral to telecare. Telecare technologies imply a spatial separation between healthcare professionals and patients in which physical contacts are replaced by virtual encounters. Following Giddens, telemedical technologies can be considered as disembedded, abstract systems in which patient–doctor relations are lifted from their local contexts and recombined across time/space distances (Giddens, 1991, p. 242). Maggie Mort and her colleagues captured this phenomenon very nicely with the terms 'remote doctors' and 'absent patients' (Mort el al., 2003). Telecare technologies thus disturb and reduce the physical proximity between healthcare providers and their patients.

To capture, and further explore, this changing spatial configuration of healthcare, I introduce the notion of technogeography of care.[6] The concept provides a useful tool for understanding how the spatial dynamics of the relationships between healthcare professionals, patients and technologies constitute specific professional and patient identities and forms of care.[7] I will use the concept to refer to two interrelated processes.

First, the notion of technogeography of care provides a useful heuristic for studying how places matter in healthcare. Although telecare technologies introduce virtual encounters between healthcare providers and patients, the use of telecare devices is always situated somewhere. In contrast to the rhetoric on telecare, which emphasizes spatially unbounded care practices, telecare technologies still largely depend on locally grounded, situated care acts. As already described above, an important place implicated in telecare technologies is the patient's home. Telecare technologies involve the relocation of healthcare from the hospital and the general practitioner's rooms to the home. Research on how home-care technologies affect patients' homes suggests that telecare technologies also play an important role in redefining the home. Studies of high-tech home-care technologies have shown how receiving long-term healthcare at home changes 'the meanings and the experience of being "at home" and "in place"' (Angus et al., 2005, p. 164; Willems, 2008, 2010; Lehoux et al., 2004). As Christine Milligan has argued, the 'reordering of the home into a space of care' involves a continuous renegotiation of the meaning of home as a site of care and a place of social relations and personal life (Milligan, 2009, p. 71, 72). Angus and colleagues explained these changes in terms of conflicts between the aesthetics and logics of healthcare and those of the home. The ambience of the home is affected by the intrusion of technological objects unfamiliar to the private space of home (Angus et al., 2005; Lehoux et al., 2004). Telecare technologies drastically extend this 'medicalization of the home' because they introduce medical devices for monitoring and diagnosing chronic diseases that occur frequently in western industrialized countries, including diabetes, respiratory insufficiency, and heart failure. Telecare technologies not only extend the medicalization of the home to a broader population; they also introduce another configuration of care. Whereas home-care technologies consisting of stand-alone medical devices require skilled nurses who pay regular visits to patients' homes to instruct and monitor patients and their informal caregivers (Arras et al., 1995, p. 3), telecare technologies delegate the responsibility for monitoring to patients. Telecare devices are expected to be used at home or in other non-clinical spaces without the presence or assistance of nurses. It is therefore important to study how patients manage to become competent users of telecare devices in the absence of skilled others. A second important difference from home-care technologies is that telecare technologies can be used to extract information electronically from the home, which redefines the notion of home as a private, physical space. Telecare technologies, and the healthcare professionals that evaluate and process these data, thus enter a place that has traditionally been protected against public officials and governmental services interfering with private family life (Brown and Webster, 2004, p. 85). I will therefore trace how these transformations of the home shape patients' relation to and use of telecare technologies.

A second place implicated in telecare technologies is the telemedical centre. Telecare technologies largely depend on these new organizations, which indeed are the very reason for their existence. The emergence of these new organizations is accompanied by the rise of a new category of healthcare professionals: telenurses and telephysicians. Telecare technologies are thus not only important in redefining identities of traditional healthcare professionals, they are key actors in creating the identity of a new kind of healthcare professional. The major work delegated to telecare professionals is that they are expected to make up for the absence of physical interaction between patients and doctors implicated in telecare technologies. This absence of physical interaction provides a major challenge to existing traditions and practices of healthcare in which proximity to patients plays a pivotal role. According to medical sociologists, sustaining a meaningful proximity to patients is a crucial aspect of healthcare (Malone, 2003). The absence of face-to-face contacts between healthcare providers and patients scripted in telecare technologies implies that healthcare professionals can only rely on images and graphs that have to speak for the patient. Techniques such as palpitation and touch, 'a cornerstone of healthcare' (Cartwright, 2000, p. 351) and literally seeing the patient are no longer available to them. An exploration of these changing spatial dimensions of the interactions between healthcare providers and patients is important in understanding how telecare technologies redefine healthcare.

Finally, telecare technologies are not only instrumental in moving care to new places; they also make certain places disappear or become less central in healthcare. The introduction of virtual encounters implies that the general practitioner's office and the hospital will be visited less frequently by patients in need of care. To understand how telecare technologies are transforming the spatial dimensions of healthcare thus requires an exploration of how places and their disappearance matter. I will use the notion of technogeography of care therefore not only as a heuristic tool, but also to intervene critically in discourses that celebrate the independence of place and time. Since the emergence of information and communication technologies, particularly the Internet, advocates of the new technologies as well as academic scholars have emphasized and celebrated the erasure of distance and place by global networks and the free flow of information and people. Like discourses on the Internet, discourses on telecare also tend to ignore place. The very name of the technology – telecare, or telemedical technology – portrays these innovations as tools that provide care-at-a-distance without specifying the places involved. This representation tends to make us believe that locations where care takes place are no longer relevant. When addressed at all, sites such as the home are presented as a 'tabula rasa' in which telecare devices can be introduced unproblematically. In this book I go beyond the view that places don't matter, a rhetoric that also slips too easily into sociological accounts of telemedicine. In their overview of studies of telemedicine, Brown and Webster, for example, describe telemedicine as 'systems of technical apparatus for abstracting bodies from the specificities of context, lifting or expropriating them from the specificities of time and place' (Brown and Webster, 2004, p. 81). Although this description may be adequate to describe the outcome of telemedical technologies, it ignores the fact that the production of data is bound to specific locations, most notably the patient's home and the telemedical centre. I therefore aim to make visible how places still matter in telecare, despite, or rather because of, the move from physical to virtual encounters between healthcare providers and patients.

A second way in which I use the notion of technnogeography of care is as a heuristic for understanding how telecare technologies create interdependencies and distribute responsibilities among people and between humans and technological objects. Whereas human geography argues that we should be sensitive to places, STS emphasize the importance of paying attention to how technologies produce specific geographies of responsibilities (Akrich, 1992). The distribution of healthcare over different places and actors inscribed in telecare technologies implies shifting responsibilities and interdependencies among patients, healthcare providers, and telecare devices. Conceptualizing these transformations in terms of changes in geography rather than network, which is the central metaphor in material–semiotic approaches to technology, particularly actor network theory, is important for drawing attention to processes in which the distribution of responsibilities takes place between actors and places that are not equally situated in healthcare. In contrast to the metaphor of a network which assumes non-hierarchical relations between humans and technological objects, the term 'geography' makes us sensitive to distributions of responsibilities which grant agency and power to specific actors while restricting or silencing the agency of others (Oudshoorn et al., 2005).

Given the vested interests of key actors in the field of telecare technology, we may expect that some places and actors will be put in the light whereas others are underrepresented in dominant discourses concerning the new technology. As feminist scholars have argued, we should be careful not to adopt too narrow an interpretation of the Latourian adage 'following the actor' to avoid the risk of reinforcing the perspectives and interests of producers and other advocates of technologies, thus silencing what is backgrounded or excluded in discourses on new technologies (Star, 1991; Clarke and Montini, 1993; Clarke 1998; Saetnan et al., 2000). The promises of telecare technologies articulated by innovators often silence the work and perspectives of major actors, particularly patients and telecare workers, although telecare technologies delegate major responsibilities to them. The research presented in this book provides a critical intervention in these discourses by rendering visible the work of these silenced actors.

Equally importantly, my account of telecare technologies addresses resistances to the new technology. Advocates of telecare technologies often argue that ambivalences and resistances towards these technologies can be understood in terms of a generational problem. Resistances are usually explained by referring to the older generation of healthcare professionals and patients who are not yet familiar with ICT-based devices. In this line of thinking, reluctant attitudes towards telecare technologies will disappear by themselves when the older generation of healthcare professionals and patients is replaced by the younger generation.[8] However, the expectation that a decrease in resistance is just a matter of time ignores reluctances that may be related to other than cognitive or behavioural differences. Adopting the material–semiotic view of technology, it seems likely that resistance to new technologies also emerges because actors do not accept the responsibilities delegated to them or others, or are not willing or able to perform the tasks delegated to them. As Akrich and Latour have argued, actors rarely comply with the actions and responsibilities inscribed in the technology; rather they negotiate, modify, resist, or bypass these scripts (Akrich, 1992; Akrich and Latour, 1992). Although technological objects can define the relationships between people and technical devices, they suggest that 'this geography is open to question and may be resisted' (Akrich, 1992, p. 207). This is an important remark because otherwise script approaches to technology may result in the very technological determinist view of technology which they were designed to avoid. Following Akrich and Latour, resistances to telecare technologies can thus be understood as resistances to the new order or form of care implicated in telecare technologies, rather than just a generational incompetency on the part of older healthcare professionals and patients.

Understanding resistances to new technologies is important because persistent ambivalences and reluctances can result in the rejection or selective use of telecare technologies that may constrain patients' access to healthcare. By focusing on selective use and non-use, I aim to contribute to the growing literature on user–technology relations in STS. Compared to users, non-users have drawn considerably less attention in this field, with a few notable exceptions (Fischer 1992; Kline and Pinch, 1996; Kline, 2000, 2003; Wyatt et al., 2002; Wyatt, 2003). This neglect of non-users is not innocent. By focusing almost exclusively on users, we may implicitly reinforce what Everett Rogers has called the 'pro-innovation bias', a view of technology that suggests that 'an innovation should be diffused and adopted by all members of a social system' (Rogers, 2003). User studies thus run the risk of contributing to a discourse which highlights adoption and use rather than rejection and discontinuance of new technologies (Rogers, 2003, p. 11). 'Pro-adoption bias' thus seems to be a better term to capture this problem.[9] In dominant policy discourses and much of the academic literature on the diffusion of technologies, non-users and users who are reluctant to adopt new technologies are framed solely in negative terms. People who choose not to use a technology are described as 'have nots' rather than as individuals who make deliberate choices concerning the use of a specific technology (Selwyn, 2003); individuals who are slow to adopt a technology are labelled as 'laggards' (Rogers, 2003); and people who stop using a technology are called 'drop-outs' (Katz and Aspden, 1998). More recently, scholars have begun to criticize this view of the adoption of new technologies in which non-use is portrayed as a deficiency and voluntary rejection does not exist. To counterbalance the narrow and often negative approaches to non-use, Sally Wyatt and colleagues introduced a conceptualization of non-use that includes the voluntary and involuntary aspects of non-use (Wyatt et al., 2002).[10] This re-conceptualization of non-users is important because it enables us to go beyond the modernist rhetoric of technological progress 'including a worldview in which adoption and use of new technologies is the norm' (Wyatt,

2003, p. 78). My account of the emerging geography of telecare will therefore also address the perspectives and care practices of voluntary and non-voluntary non-users of telecare devices.

Research questions, method and organization of the book

To conclude, the major aim of this book is to understand how telecare technologies challenge existing healthcare and create new geographies of care. How do telecare technologies participate in reordering healthcare? Which forms of care are created? What kinds of healthcare professionals and patients are constituted in this changing landscape of care? To answer these questions I adopt a multi-sited approach to investigate the implementation and use of three different telecare devices for heart patients introduced in the US and Europe (particularly in Germany and the Netherlands): a telecare system for heart-failure patients, a heart mobile phone for assisting patients at risk of heart attacks, and a telecare device to diagnose heart-rhythm irregularities. These telecare devices represent different phases in the life trajectory of technologies: the heart mobile phone and the device for diagnosing heart rhythm have been on the market since the mid-1990s, whereas the telemonitoring system for heart-failure patients was introduced ten years later. Moreover, the telecare devices are introduced by medical companies with a different track record in this sector. The monitoring system for heart-failure was introduced in the US by Philips, a large, multinational electronics firm that is a relative newcomer to the field of telemonitoring technologies, and implemented in the Netherlands by the same company in collaboration with a major Dutch health insurer, Achmea. The heart mobile phone was introduced in several European countries by Vitaphone, a medium-sized firm in Germany specializing in various telecare devices and the owner of a telemedical centre. The diagnostic device for heart-rhythm disturbances was put on the market in the Netherlands and Germany by Hartis B. V., a small Dutch company that runs a telemedical centre and has no other products. This variety in devices, firms, and national contexts enables me study the dynamics of the implementation and use of telecare devices for heart patients implemented in healthcare during the past decade. I track and trace the multiple sites and actors involved in these novel healthcare practices and describe how these telecare devices have contributed to the reordering of healthcare and the creation of new professional and patient identities.[11]

The design of this book is as follows. Part I, *Reordering Care*, focuses on how telecare technologies challenge and redefine the order of healthcare. The chapters in this section describe the redistribution of tasks and responsibilities of healthcare work implicated in telecare technologies and the resistances to this reordering of care. Chapter 3 focuses on the promises articulated by producers and implementers of telecare technologies about what these technologies contribute to healthcare. I analyse the problems innovators promise to solve, what roles they define, and for whom. This chapter describes how innovators paint a rather rosy future for the new technology and examines the places, actors, and perspectives that are silenced in these accounts of telecare devices for heart patients. Chapter 4 addresses the resistance of healthcare professionals to the emerging geography of telecare. The chapter describes how the introduction of telecare technologies disturbs the order of care: it challenges the professional autonomy of healthcare professionals because tasks previously allocated to them are partly delegated to telecare workers. Adopting the concept of boundary work, the chapter shows how healthcare professionals contest and resist this reordering of care to maintain their professional authority. These contestations about 'who cares?' not only shape the boundaries of the new profession of telecare workers but also redefine the identity of users and the technology itself.

Part II of the book, *Creating New Forms of Care*, focuses on how telecare technologies transform the places, the work and the care practices of healthcare professionals. Chapter 5 describes how the introduction of telecare technologies has resulted in the creation of new spaces for providing healthcare: telemedical centres, staffed by telecare workers. The chapter traces the emergence of telemedical centres and describes how the healthcare work provided in these novel spaces is largely defined by the scripts of ICT devices, which constitute telecare as highly pre-structured, protocol-driven work. The kind of healthcare professional created in telemedical centres is a healthcare provider who is disciplined in prioritizing the objective, standardized knowledge inscribed in telecare devices over their own practical knowledge. The chapter shows how telecare workers do not passively follow these scripts but often rely on their experiential and tacit knowledge to provide healthcare according to their own standards of care. Chapter 6 continues the analysis of the changing spatial dimensions of care by comparing healthcare services for heart patients based on face-to-face contacts with healthcare delivered remotely. This chapter analyses what kinds of knowledge and care are created, valued, and neglected in healthcare based on physical contacts between healthcare providers and patients in a polyclinic compared to remote consultations mediated by a telemedical centre.

The chapter shows how places matter in defining healthcare by describing how polyclinics and telemedical centres constitute different kinds of care. Whereas polyclinics facilitate contextualized, personal healthcare, telemedical centres support individualized, immediate healthcare. Part III of the book, *Redefining Patients and Home*, addresses the question of how telecare technologies participate in transforming the identities of patients and redefining the home. Although patients are often absent in discourses on telecare technologies and the patient's home emerges as a tabula rasa, these technologies introduce a new healthcare practice in which patients are expected to play an active role by inspecting their own bodies. Chapter 7 examines the invisible work it takes to produce patients who are active and responsible as participants in the diagnosis of heart problems. The chapter describes how telecare devices define patients as diagnostic agents, create interdependencies between patients and healthcare professionals, and redefine patients' home and public spaces. Chapter 8 extends the investigation of how telecare technologies change patients' identities and homes by including non-users of telecare devices in the analysis. This chapter compares and contrasts the experiences and practices of users and non-users of telecare devices and describes how participation in these different technology-mediated care practices constitutes different ways of inspecting the body and coping with disease. The chapter shows how the use of telecare devices at home has changed the relationships between body, technology, self, and close relatives, a transformation rejected by non-users. The concluding chapter, finally, evaluates the major conclusions that one can draw from this account of the implementation and use of telecare technologies and their implications for policy and design.

Part I
Reordering Care

3
Promises, Scenarios, and Silences

> Novel technologies do not substantively pre-exist them-
> selves except only in terms of the imaginings, expecta-
> tions and visions that have shaped their potential.
>
> (Borup et al., 2006, p. 285)

Technologies cannot exist without promises. Biographies of technologies are therefore fascinating to read because they often describe expectations and promises that are no longer part of our collective memory
or else have become part and parcel, the 'essence', of the technology
as we know it today. Although promises thus may come and go, they
are never innocent. The field of science and technology studies (STS)
has a rich literature, which indicates that expectations play an important role in the development of technologies. One of the important
insights of studies of the sociology of expectations, one of the themes
in STS, is that promises can be considered as 'wishful enactments of a
desired future' (Borup et al., 2006, p. 286). Expectations are not merely
rhetorical but 'constitutive' or 'performative' in attracting the interest
and mobilizing the support of actors considered necessary to make the
technologies work, such as other innovators, investors, policymakers,
and users (Borup et al., 2006, p. 289). Expectations not only define the
relevant actors, they also allocate specific roles to them as well as to the
(future) technology. Expectations are thus understood as containing a
script or scenario of the future world (Lente and Rip, 1998, p. 203). This
scenario specifies how people and things should act and is, in this sense,
obligatory: it is 'an implicit warrant to others that they should use that
tool or procedure' (Borup et al., 2006, p. 289).

Although these studies provide useful insights into the role of
expectations in technological development, they are largely restricted

to understanding how expectations and promises shape the early development of technologies within Research & Development (R&D) departments in industry and academia.[1] I suggest it is relevant to study promises in a later phase of technological development, after artefacts have left the R&D departments to become part of the world outside the laboratories. This shift in focus is important because studies in the sociology of expectations tend to camouflage the risks, anxieties, and other social/cultural processes that may constrain technological innovation.[2] This absence can be ascribed partly to the fact that negative expectations are often not articulated in the early phases of technological development. To attract the interest of relevant actors, early promises tend to paint a rather rosy future of the technology and often contain utopian, technology-driven dreams about how the world would look if everyone were to use the new technology. Or, as the historian Marvin put it, every age tends to 'read the future as a fancier version of the present' (Marvin, 1988). Moreover, early promises tend to downplay the cultural and organizational processes on which the future of a technology depends (Borup et al., 2006, p. 290), which may explain their absence from the sociology of expectations. However, the fact that anxieties and socio-cultural aspects are understudied can also be ascribed to the research agenda in a field that focuses on understanding how expectations shape R&D practices and science policies. Adopting the view that promises are important not only in shaping R&D but also in trying to define future use, I think it is important to study both positive and negative expectations and, when the latter are not articulated, to analyse the absences and silences in these discourses. Which actors, roles, perspectives, and concerns have no voice in expectation statements?

In this chapter I investigate the promises made about what telecare technologies will contribute to healthcare. Adopting the techno-geographical approach introduced in the previous chapter, my aim is to give voice to silenced actors, places, and perspectives implicated in the new technologies. How and to what extent are changes in the landscape of care, in terms of a redistribution of responsibilities between people, places, and technological devices and the changing meanings of places where care takes place, represented in the promises?In my analysis I address the following questions:

1 What problems in healthcare do innovators promise to solve? What scenarios about healthcare are articulated in promises about telecare technologies?

2 What roles are defined, and for whom and what? Who is expected to care for and with telecare technologies?

3 Whose needs and worries are addressed? Whose perspectives on care and illness are taken into account?

4 Which actors, roles, places, and perspectives on which the future of technologies depend are silenced?

To study the promises and silences in expectation statements articulated during the introduction and use of telecare technologies I analyse the websites of producers, press bulletins that announce the clinical testing and implementation of telecare devices, and brochures to promote the new technology among healthcare professionals in the US and Europe. Websites, press bulletins, and brochures play an important role in the articulation and circulation of promises. I focus on promises related to the three telecare devices for heart patients that are the central focus in this book: a telemonitoring system for heart-failure patients, a heart mobile phone for assisting patients at risk of heart attacks, and a telemonitoring device to diagnose heart-rhythm irregularities. The next three sections analyse these promises. The chapter concludes with a summary of and reflection on the absences and silences in promises on telecare technologies and how these are addressed in the following chapters.

Telemonitoring device for heart-failure patients

Problems and scenario

Technologies to monitor heart failure at a distance are a very recent innovation. In the US, the first telemonitoring system was put on the market in 2006; one year later, the same technology was introduced in Europe, in the Netherlands, and clinical studies were initiated in Germany. This new telecare technology was introduced by Philips, one of the largest electronics companies in the world with market leadership positions in diagnostic imaging and patient telecare technologies as well as electronic technologies for consumers such as TV. Philips is a relative newcomer to the market of telecare technologies, devices that extend the reach of care to locations outside the hospital and the physician's rooms. Their telemonitoring system for heart failure, called Motiva, is the company's first telecare system. It consists of wireless devices for the daily measurement of weight and blood pressure. These measurements, collected by patients at home, are automatically sent to a telemedical centre (in the Netherlands) or a hospital (in the US) (see Figure 3.1).

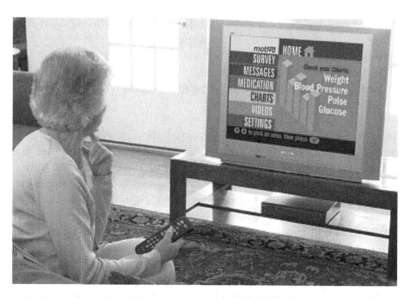

Figure 3.1   TV screen of the heart-failure monitoring system

In case of deviant measures, the telemonitoring system signals nurses who phone patients to ask them why they have failed to keep their weight and blood pressure within the set standards. When the system uses a telemedical centre, telenurses inform nurses at the hospital who have the authority to change medication or to organize a visit to the polyclinic or the cardiologist. (Balk et al., 2007, p. 56).

Philips put quite some effort into articulating and circulating their promises about this new technology by launching various press releases. The first press bulletin appeared in the autumn of 2004 to announce that the company had begun a pilot study of the new technology in Andover, Massachusetts, US, to test usability and adoption among patients and healthcare providers (Philips, press information, 2004). In subsequent years, the firm also informed the press about other events such as the results of the pilot study and the commercial launch of the technology in 2006. The pilot study was also announced on the company's website. From 2005, Philips also tried to stimulate interest in this new technology among European audiences and began to inform the press about the launch of their first European pilot study, for which they had chosen the Netherlands. The aim of this study was to 'quantify the impact of the new technology on overall quality of care' (Philips, press information, 2005). Information about this study was also posted on the company's website and the website of Achmea, the healthcare insurance company that financed the study and is the owner of the telemedical centre involved in its testing. Achmea is one of the largest health insurers in the Netherlands and part of a leading insurance group operating in several other European countries (Philips, press information, 2004).

A closer look at these press releases and websites shows that Philips and Achmea are rather consistent in the promises they articulate about the telecare technology. All sources mention by and large the same positive expectations, although not always in the same order or with the same priorities. One major promise articulated in the press releases and the webpages is that telecare technologies will reduce the costs of healthcare, described as one of the biggest problems in current and future healthcare. The telemonitoring system for heart-failure is portrayed as a tool that can help healthcare organizations to deliver care at a lower cost. This promise is usually accompanied by calculations of healthcare budgets spent on chronic patients, particularly patients suffering from cardiovascular diseases. Jay Mazelsky, general manager of the new ventures business unit for Philips Medical Systems, described this problem in the press release that announced the pilot study in the US:

> In the United States, approximately 78 percent of healthcare spending is on chronic conditions. In fact, cardiovascular disease – the number one killer in the United States – costs over \$225 billion per year. This includes congestive heart failure, the leading cause of hospital admissions for people over 65, which afflicts about 5 million patients.
>
> (Philips, press information, 2004)

In the press information for the European market, the company expresses a similar concern with costs. Philips, now joined by the Dutch healthcare insurer Achmea, presented the new technology as 'a cost-effective way for European healthcare'.[3] This promise was also articulated on Achmea's website[4] and emphasized by the senior managers of the health insurer (interview Helm and Boutkan, 2006; interview Leussen, 2007). The reduction of costs is thus a central concern in the promises articulated around this new technology.

The press releases not only address the economic and efficiency concerns of healthcare organizations but also include promises to patients. The telemonitoring system will not only reduce costs, it will also contribute to improving the quality of life and empowering patients.[5] These promises are not articulated separately but in relation to the promises about productivity and cost reduction. Philips press releases and web-pages often include sentences in which these promises are closely intertwined:

> Through advanced, easy-to-use remote patient management technology, such as Motiva, Philips aims to improve the productivity of healthcare providers and empower patients to take a more active role in managing their own health. This in turn can help healthcare organizations deliver more effective care at a lower cost.
>
> (Philips, press information, 2004)

This coupling of promises is often described as a 'win-win' situation: telecare technologies can reduce the costs of healthcare and simultaneously improve the quality of life and empower patients (Royal Philips Electronics, 2008). The promises concerning quality of life are usually formulated in terms of the contribution telecare technologies will make in reducing the risk of emergency admissions to hospital because the technology enables healthcare professionals to intervene earlier in cases where heart-failure problems are likely to get worse. Early intervention can be realized because patients are able to measure vital signs (weight and blood pressure) themselves daily at home. According to the expectation statements, this active role of patients in 'managing' their diseases contributes to the empowerment of patients (Philips, press information, 2004). The active involvement of patients will also improve so-called patient compliance. Telecare technologies will assist patients to adhere to the bodily regimen of medication, diet and exercise prescribed to them by healthcare professionals. The name of the telemonitoring system, Motiva, is carefully chosen to express this promise: Motiva will motivate patients to modify their behaviour in order to prevent a sudden worsening of their health condition (Philips, press information, 2004).

The promises articulated in the press releases and webpages imply the following scenario for healthcare. Healthcare providers and policymakers can reduce the rising costs of healthcare by implementing telecare technologies that will make care for chronic heart-failure patients more cost-effective and efficient. Patients should become more active in their own healthcare by using telecare devices. The use of the new technology will empower patients, improve their quality of life, and enhance the quality of their care. In this scenario, healthcare as we know it today will partly cease to exist and be replaced by novel ways of caring for chronic patients. The press releases and webpages clearly emphasize that telecare technologies will change the face of healthcare. Phrases such as 'paving the way to a new care model' (Philips, press information, 2004) and 'telecare technologies will change the whole way healthcare is delivered' (Philips website, 2005) are important ingredients of the expectation statements.

These changes include the introduction of virtual encounters between doctors and patients, the introduction of 'continuous monitoring and care', the extension of care to the homes of patients (described as 'bringing it all back home'), and a 'paradigm shift' in healthcare from individual-based to population-based care by connecting large populations (10,000 to 100,000) to telemonitoring systems (Interview Weijde, 2006).

Actors and roles

The promises articulated in press bulletins and webpages thus include a scenario about how telecare technologies will shape healthcare. Like other scenarios, this vision of future care specifies the actors who and roles which will realize these promises. The question thus emerges about what roles are defined in this scenario and for whom or what? Who is expected to care for and with this telecare technology? The expectation statements of Philips and Achmea are very explicit about the actors required to fulfil the promises. All the actors we might expect to find when new technologies are introduced in healthcare figure here, the one more prominently than the other, in the press releases and webpages. The expectation statements allocate roles to traditional healthcare professionals (physicians, clinicians, and nurses) and organizations (hospitals), to a new category of healthcare professionals (healthcare workers at telemedical centres) and a novel intermediary healthcare organization (the telemedical centre), to patients, and to the technology.

Let us first take a closer look at the roles allocated to healthcare professionals. In the press release that announced the pilot study of the heart-failure telemonitoring system in the US cardiovascular physicians figure most prominently. The role allocated to physicians is very straightforward; they are expected, and have agreed, to conduct the pilot study that will test how well patients will use the new technology and whether healthcare professionals will be willing and able to adapt to this new healthcare service (Philips, press information, 2004). The pilot study thus also reveals another role for physicians: they are expected not only to conduct the study but also to adopt the role of test subjects. 'Care staff' (an explanation of which healthcare professionals are implied here is not included) are expected to use the Motiva system during the period of the test and to report on their experiences (Philips, press information, 2004). The announcement of the pilot study in the US on the Philips website allocates a third role to physicians: they are expected to 'manage the condition of chronically ill patients once they have been discharged from hospital' supported by the new telecare technology (Philips website, downloaded November 25 2005). This last role is also frequently mentioned in the press releases in Europe and on the Philips website (Achmea and Philips press information, 2005). Physicians are thus considered as crucial actors in the scenario for healthcare. They have to act as testers, test-subjects, and healthcare providers willing to adapt their current care practices to the new technology.

Compared to physicians, nurses figure less prominently in the expectation statements in the US. Press releases announcing the pilot study in the US refer to nurses only implicitly when they mention the role of 'care staff'. In the press releases announcing the first pilot study in Europe, nurses figure more prominently. This press information allocates roles to two categories of nurse: telenurses who work in the telemedical centre run by Achmea, and heart-failure nurses who work at the polyclinic of the involved hospitals. Telenurses are expected to 'monitor the patients' health and support them by sending reminder messages and educational videos, responding to inbound patient phone calls, and performing triage if medical attention is needed' (Achmea and Philips, press information, 2005). Heart-failure nurses, who receive less attention, are presented as actors who will be contacted by telenurses 'when measurements are beyond the normal range' (Achmea and Philips, press information, 2005). The absence of telenurses from press information about the US pilot study can be ascribed to the fact that in the US the telemonitoring system is connected directly to healthcare professionals in the hospital. In this respect, the scenario for healthcare in the US differs from the scenario in Europe, where telenurses and telemedical centres figure as important new intermediary actors and institutions in future healthcare. In the press information that announced the European pilot study, the telemedical centre is portrayed as an important actor for fulfilling the promises of the new technology.

A third group of actors expected to play a role in realizing the promises of the new technology are the patients. The first role allocated to patients is that of mere users. In the expectation statements in the press releases of the pilot study and the commercial launch in the US patients are addressed only as users of the new technology. The emphasis is not so much on how the technology may help them to cope with their diseases but on the user-friendliness of the technology. Patients are expected to use the telemonitoring system to measure vital signs such as weight and blood pressure and to watch educational videos and graphs of the measurements on TV (Philips, press information, 2004) (see Figure 3.1 and 3.2). The press information emphasizes that patients easily integrate the new technology into their daily routines because they have only to 'spend a few minutes each day at their convenience interacting with Motiva' (Philips, press information, 2006). A second, related role allocated to patients is that they are expected to 'modify their behavior', which implies that they should 'follow their doctor's guidelines, eat right, and exercise more' (Philips, press information, 2005) with the help of the new technology. The use of telecare technology will not only affect patients' individual behaviour but also change their relationship with healthcare professionals:

> With Motiva, patients interact with their healthcare provider ... supporting a stronger personal relationship between patient and provider that is intended to deepen the commitment to improving self-care.
>
> (Achmea website, 2005)

In this press release, the active role allocated to patients is thus rephrased in terms of 'self-care'. A similar role is described in one of

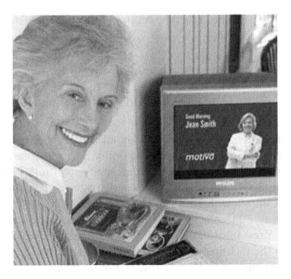

Figure 3.2 Female user of the heart-failure telemonitoring system

Philips's promotional brochures, which portrays patients as 'managers' of their disease. To articulate the role of patients, press releases sometimes include photos of patients, often the same picture showing an elderly woman who seems fairly healthy and relaxed while using a blood-pressure meter or watching an educational video on TV in her living room (Achmea and Philips press information, 2005).

The photos are in sharp contrast to some of the textual information about patients, which suggests that heart-failure patients are not so healthy because they often suffer from multiple chronic diseases (Philips website, 25 November 2005). Patients are represented not only by pictures; their voices are also sometimes included in the press releases or webpages. One press release quoted a patient named Bobby DiSipio as follows:

> Just as the name suggests, Motiva motivated me to do the right thing. Through personal charts and educational videos sent to me on my TV by my nurse, I learned how to better manage my disease. I weighed myself, took my own blood pressure, answered daily health questions, and the Motiva system tracked how well I was doing. With Motiva, it was easy to learn how improving my lifestyle could help me stay healthier. I'm feeling more in control now.
>
> (Philips, press information, 2005)

In another press release, a participant in the US pilot study described his experience as follows:

> If you know how to press a button, you know how it operates. The TV screen tells you everything you need to do.
>
> (Philips, press information, 2006)

Although patients are expected to play an active role in the scenario of healthcare, their roles, except in the quotes above, are expressed in the passive voice: 'patients will receive a remote control' (Philips, press information, 2004), 'Motiva will help patients to manage their disease' (Philips website, downloaded on 25 November 2005), 'Motiva enables people to play a more active role in managing their health' (Achmea and Philips, press information, 2005), all statements in which agency is allocated to the technology rather than the patient.

Finally, the scenario for healthcare not only articulates roles for human actors but also describes roles for the technology itself. In the press releases and webpages important roles and agencies are delegated to the telemonitoring system. The overall role ascribed to the technology is to motivate patients to change their behaviour. This role is further specified in three sub-roles. The technology is expected to deliver healthcare information and educational videos to patients; to provide feedback to patients in order to encourage a healthy lifestyle; and to connect patients to their healthcare provider (Philips, press information, 2004). The technology is thus expected to play a pivotal role in realizing the scenario for healthcare: it orders and creates links between healthcare professionals and patients.

Perspectives and silences

Although the scenario for healthcare articulated in the promises of the innovators allocates roles to all relevant actors, including the technology, this does not imply that all actors are represented in a similar manner. The expectation statements illustrate that the perspectives of some actors are foregrounded whereas the perspectives of others receive less attention or are silenced. The most dominant perspective expressed in the press releases and webpages is the managerial view of care, a view primarily concerned with the costs of healthcare or other management problems, such as productivity and efficiency concerns (Royal Philips Electronics, 2008). This perspective is clearly reflected in the name sometimes used to refer to the technology: 'a home-based management solution' (Philips, press information, 2004). This managerial view is linked to the economic interests of Philips and, in the Netherlands, Achmea. On the Philips webpages, the company explains its involvement in the development and introduction of telecare technologies for chronic patients in terms of 'brand fidelity':

> The improvement of the quality of life of chronic patients is one of the ways to realize brand fidelity. By doing this we strengthen our position as a healthcare, lifestyle and technology company. This is also the driving force behind the new interactive Motiva-platform for communication in healthcare.
>
> (Philips website, 2005)

Philips's perspective on healthcare is thus explicitly linked to the company's endeavour to improve its position in the healthcare market, which they consider the biggest growth market for the company in the near future. For several years Philips has tried hard to profile itself as a company that delivers healthcare technologies, which included the take-over of several medical companies. The announcement of the first European pilot study triggered the interest of stockmarket actors, including the Dow Jones News Service, who expected that the firm would increase its share rates (Grinsven, 2005). Like Philips, Achmea also follows clear economic incentives that are included in the expectation statements. The healthcare insurance company expects a reduction in costs of healthcare to improve its competitive position in relation to other health insurance companies in the Netherlands.

Compared to the innovators' perspectives, the perspectives of healthcare providers and patients receive less emphasis in the expectation statements, or are mentioned only in a very specific way. Healthcare professionals are clearly represented in the expectation statements, sometimes by using quotations. These representations are, however, restricted to the cardiologists in charge of the coordination of the pilot studies, the so-called 'principal investigators' (Philips press information, 2004). These experiences thus reflect a researchers' rather than a healthcare providers' perspective. The views of 'ordinary' healthcare providers on whether they think that the new technology will improve current care for chronic patients, or whether they are willing to adopt the new technology in their hospital, is missing from the press information and webpages. Also absent is any reference to the ways in which telecare technologies will change the current distribution of tasks and responsibilities, and whether healthcare professionals will be willing to collaborate with telecare professionals, and vice versa.

Like healthcare professionals' perspectives, patients' perspectives are represented in a very restricted manner. Promises often refer to abstract notions such as improvement of the 'quality of life' or statistics on the reduction of the frequency of hospital admissions. Although patients are sometimes quoted, these quotes merely represent a functionalistic perspective on how the technology affects patients' lives, describing how the technology enables a patient to 'manage his disease', or 'how he felt more in control by using the technology' (Philips, press information, 2005) (patients are thus referred to as male) or how easy it was to use the system (Achmea website, 2005). The only time a broader patients perspective was included was in an expectation statement by a Philips manager, who described how patients prefer to live at home, want to remain independent, and often suffer from multiple chronic diseases (Philips website, downloaded 25 November 2005). Questions about whether patients are willing to become 'managers' of their disease (Philips, press information, 2004) or how the use of telecare devices will change the meaning of home or being a heart patient are not addressed in the expectation statements.

The heart mobile phone: Telemonitoring of heart attacks

Problems and scenario

Although cellphones have been available for general communication purposes for almost two decades, the exchange of electrocardiograms (ECGs) by mobile phone is a more recent innovation. An ECG is a representation of the electrical activity of the heart in the form of a strip graph. ECGs are widely used in the detection and diagnosis of cardiovascular diseases. ECG signals are well suited to transmission by phone because they can easily be converted into an audible tone (Moore, 1999, p. 252). The first ECG-recording cellphone, or so-called Herz Handy (heart mobile phone) was introduced in Germany in 1999 by the German firm Vitaphone founded that same year. In 2003 the heart mobile phone was made available to Swiss citizens by a Swiss subsidiary of the German company and Austrian citizens (interview Sack, 2004). In the same period, two Dutch entrepreneurs were permitted to use the name Vitaphone to introduce the new technology into the Netherlands.[6] Currently, the German company employs approximately 50 staff and provides various mobile phones and digital cards for safety and health purposes, including mobile phones for the elderly, emergency cellphones, and the heart mobile phone.[7] The heart mobile phone, claimed to be 'the world's first mobile phone that is capable of recording, storing and transmitting an ECG',[8] was designed by the German cardiologist Stefan Sack, one of the founders of Vitaphone, and manufactured by the Finnish tele-communication company Benefon (Interview Quinger, 2004). The heart mobile phone consists of an ECG-recording cellphone that can be used by heart patients outdoors. When they experience heart problems, they have to remove the back side of the shell of the phone to display the four ECG electrodes, put the back side of the phone to the left side of their bare chest, call the telemedical centre and press buttons to record and send an ECG to the centre. Healthcare staff at the telemedical centre will answer the phone, analyse the ECG, instruct the patient what he/she should do, and forward the data to the treating physician. In the case of an emergency, telecare professionals can ask the nearest rescue service to send an ambulance, facilitated by the mobile heart phone's global positioning system (GPS) that can provide the exact location of the caller, with an accuracy of 15 metres.[9]

To promote the new technology to potential customers, Vitaphone has developed a very extensive (60-page), well-designed website,[10] including text, images, graphics and animations, and brochures with pictures and detailed descriptions of the telecare devices that can be downloaded from the website. The major promise articulated on the website is that the heart mobile phone will provide heart patients with increased safety and mobility in their daily lives by monitoring their heart conditions:

> Each year 350,000 people die from heart attack in Germany. Another 80,000 cases of sudden cardiac death only adds to this tragic balance. Heart attack survivors live in constant fear of experiencing further life-threatening heart and circulation problems. Being alone, without immediate aid in the case of sudden heart or circulation problems is a cause for great anxiety. With the heart mobile phone Vitaphone provides heart patients with an individual solution for more safety and mobility in their everyday lives, a solution that leads to a considerable improvement in their quality of life.[11]

The text is accompanied by a picture of a man fishing together with a boy, presumably his grandson. This promise is highlighted in the company's headpiece that appears on each webpage: 'Vitaphone, Safety & Mobility'. The web pages repeat the promise that the heart mobile phone can assist in saving the lives of heart patients by providing prompt aid, using phrases such as: 'help is always just a press of a button away', or 'you will never be alone'.[12] The latter phrase is used to explain that the heart mobile phone enables heart patients to access immediate care even during vacations or in remote places.

In contrast to Philips's expectation statements, the promises articulated on Vitaphone's website largely focus on patients. Promises addressing healthcare professionals are not included in the first 20 pages of the website but only included in the section entitled 'The company and Telemedicine'. This difference in priorities reflects a different marketing strategy. Whereas Philips considers healthcare professionals as their major target group (the heart-failure monitoring system is sold to hospitals), Vitaphone, at least on their website, primarily addresses patients who are considered as major clients of the company. Vitaphone's website is not only a tool to circulate promises and attract the attention of patients or healthcare professionals, it also functions as a sales instrument: patients can order a heart mobile phone off the website. However, healthcare professionals remain an important target group for Vitaphone as well. The company had to modify its original business model based on targeting individual consumers to a business model that delivers the mobile phone as a technology prescribed by physicians,[13] and this dual strategy is reflected in the company's website. Although promises to patients dominate the website, promises to healthcare organizations and professionals are also articulated. The use of the heart mobile phone and other Vitaphone products will lead to 'medium-term cost reductions' and 'improved quality of care'.[14]

Similar promises are articulated in the glossy brochure on the heart mobile phone that is clearly targeted to healthcare professionals. The brochure text promises that 'the companies pioneering e-Health concepts' and 'key technologies' will contribute to 'improving diagnostics, therapy and patient management' and deliver a 'life-saving emergency management'.[15] The brochure also includes promises to healthcare organizations, that is, that Vitaphone's products and services will contribute to saving costs without reducing the quality of care.[16] Like Philips, Vitaphone does not restrict its promises to current healthcare but claims that its products will be instrumental in 'defining the medicine of the future'.[17]

Vitaphone's website and brochure describe the following scenario for healthcare. Patients can be less anxious about their heart because the heart mobile phone provides immediate access to medical care. The telemonitoring device will save lives, reduce the time spent in hospital and rehabilitation, and enhance the mobility of patients. Healthcare professionals and policymakers can solve financial problems and improve the quality of care because the new technology will make healthcare more cost-effective and improve the quality of diagnostics, therapy, and medical care.

Actors and roles

In the promises articulated in the website and the brochure, Vitaphone puts quite some effort into defining the actors and roles required to realize the scenario of life-saving, high-quality, and cost-effective healthcare provision. As might be expected, a first major group of actors defined in the scenario are patients. Patients figure very prominently on the website, although they receive less attention in the brochure. The role allocated to patients is an active one in healthcare.[18] They have to purchase a mobile heart phone, carry it with them wherever they go, and place it on their chest whenever they experience heart problems. Most importantly, the use of the heart mobile phone is not restricted to people who survived heart attacks but also includes 'at-risk patients', individuals who have a higher chance of a heart attack than others. By including this category of patients, the number of potential users of the heart mobile phone is considerably increased. In contrast to the heart-failure telemonitoring system, the heart mobile phone does not allocate other roles to its users. The heart mobile phone is meant only to record ECGs to detect heart attacks and not as a device to discipline patients to adhere to medication or lifestyle instructions.

To articulate the role of patients, the website includes pictures of a man with his hand on his left chest (suggesting that he is experiencing heart problems), a close-up photo of the chest of a man who holds the heart mobile phone on his chest (see Figure 3.3), a picture of a man fishing with his grandson (described above), and a photo of a man running into the sea accompanied by his wife.

The pictures thus reflect the promise that heart patients can remain active outdoors without fear because they can ask for immediate medical care when they need it. The website also includes so-called case studies that contain a short video of a man experiencing a heart attack while running in a nature area. It shows how he uses the heart mobile phone to ask for medical assistance.[19] Like the photos, the video illustrates Vitaphone's promise that the use of the heart mobile phone will enable heart patients to remain mobile and active, even in

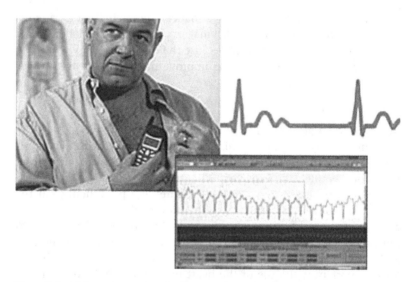

Figure 3.3 Male patient using the heart mobile phone

remote places. Whereas the website shows pictures of men only, thus suggesting that only men are at risk of a heart attack, the brochure also portrays women. The cover page shows a picture of an elderly, sporty and healthy-looking woman walking in the middle of a group of people of different ages, obviously representing her family, including two children, her husband, and two grand-daughters. A close-up of the woman's face and one of her granddaughters is used as background on the page with the table of contents. The brochure thus clearly addresses women as target groups for the heart mobile phone, which may reflect the recent shift in healthcare in which heart attacks are no longer considered as a typically male disease.

Although Vitaphone puts some effort into portraying potential users, information about how people experience the use of the heart mobile phone is missing in the website and the brochure. Quotes from interviews with patients, or references to the results of research among users of the new technology, are not included in this information. The company is, however, convinced that patients will be willing to use the heart mobile phone. Referring to a study conducted by 'the respected US management consultants Frost & Sullivan', the brochure text informs the reader that 'in Europe alone in 2011 over four million heart patients will own mobile devices that monitor their heart rates and are connected to a medical service center'.[20]

A second group of actors expected to play an important role in realizing the promises of the new technology are the healthcare professionals who work at the telemedical centres. On the website, the Vitaphone Service Center, as the telemedical centre is called, has a dominant position. Under the headline 'The Vitaphone Service Center – a platform for up to date disease management', the website introduces the telemedical centre as 'the crucial hub in all Vitaphone's eHealth services' and describes its staff as 'a competent and highly specialized team of internists and cardiologists, as well as qualified medical assistants'.[21] The tasks delegated to this team are not described extensively on the website. The text mentions only that the caller will be addressed personally and that the healthcare professionals who receive the phone call will use an electronic patient file. To illustrate how the telemedical centre looks, the website shows two pictures of six people sitting in pairs opposite each other at desks, watching computer screens and wearing headphones. In the brochure, the tasks delegated to the staff of the telemedical centre are explained in more detail, which is obviously considered important in convincing the traditional healthcare providers targeted in the brochure of the quality of this newcomer to the field of healthcare. Like the website, the brochure text emphasizes the medical expertise of the staff of the telemedical centre by describing them as 'qualified medical assistants' and doctors. The healthcare professionals at Vitaphone's Medical Service Centre are expected to look after patients; to monitor, evaluate, and document ECGs; to call an ambulance in case of emergency calls; and to give advice or instructions on first aid to patients or their next of kin. Telecare professionals are also expected to be 'familiar with the patients' medical histories'.[22] The brochure emphasizes that the telemedical centre's staff will be available '24 hours a day, 365 days a year'.

In contrast to the telecare professionals, the tasks of the traditional healthcare professionals are not addressed.[23] Their role in the scenario is described only in passive terms that explain how Vitaphone will support them with 'the best possible care for their chronically ill patients and their next of kin' and 'by improving diagnostics, therapy and patient management'.[24] The only task explicitly mentioned in the brochure is that the attending physician decides in each case whether medical intervention is required and, if so, what sort.[25] Moreover, healthcare professionals are expected to collaborate with Vitaphone to develop the company's technologies and services.[26]

Last but not least, the scenario also delegates a major role to the heart mobile phone. The role ascribed to this telemonitoring device is to save the lives of patients experiencing symptoms of a heart attack and to increase their mobility and quality of life. The way in which the heart mobile phone is presented is significant. In contrast to Philips, Vitaphone presents the heart mobile phone not as a separate device but as part of a technological network, including the telemedical centre.[27]

Described as 'the heart of the innovative telecare service concept', the telemedical centre receives even more attention than the heart mobile phone. The brochure text adopts a similar strategy by first introducing the telemedical centre as 'the core of Vitaphone's eHealthcare systems' and then describing the heart mobile phone and the other products provided by the company.[28] The heart mobile phone is thus presented not as a stand-alone product but as an actant in the telecare service developed and provided by the company. This foregrounding of the telemedical centre can be ascribed to the fact that the company is the owner and runs the centre, which explains why Vitaphone puts more emphasis on this novel intermediary healthcare organization than Philips, which does not own a telemedical centre. Vitaphone thus not only tries to sell the heart mobile phone but also aims to attract users of its telemedical centre. The brochure emphasizes that 'only a professional and coordinated combination of these elements turns new technologies into a valuable – and useful-eHealth service'.[29]

Perspectives and silences

Reflecting on the promises concerning the heart mobile phone, we can conclude that all the actors we might expect to contribute to realizing the scenario are described on the website and in the brochure. Similarly to the scenario of the heart-failure telemonitoring system, the perspectives of some actors are, however, prioritized over others, with remarkable differences between the website and the brochure. Because the website is primarily, but not exclusively, targeted at patients, their perspectives receive more attention than those of healthcare professionals. The promises as well as the ways in which the products and services are described are clearly written from the perspective of patients. The home page opens with a section 'Welcome to Vitaphone', which directly addresses patients: 'Our products let you take an active role in your healthcare.'[30] The webpage explaining the heart mobile phone also adopts the perspective of patients by describing the anxiety 'heart attack survivors' experience, particularly when they are alone without access to medical care. The video also explicitly adopts patients' perspectives. It shows how the heart mobile phone can be integrated into daily life activities and enable patients to remain active outdoors without worrying too much about their hearts. The website also contains a section for Frequently Asked Questions about the use of the heart mobile phone (May I use it outside Germany? Is it very difficult to record an ECG'? What does GPS mean?, etc.) and the telemedical centre (When can I call? Who evaluates the ECGs? Can mistakes occur during transmissions? etc.). It also contains a section 'All about the heart' that explains in biology textbook language the functioning of the heart, heart disorders, the risk factors involved in cardiovascular diseases, and how patients can protect their health. Although Vitaphone tries to adopt the perspective of patients, the information remains largely restricted to an instrumental view of the new technology and heart disorders. Questions about how patients experience the use of the heart mobile phone, at home and in public spaces, are not addressed.

In contrast to the website, the brochure is mainly targeted at healthcare professionals. This does not imply, however, that it addresses their perspectives explicitly: healthcare professionals do not figure often in the brochure. The major aim of the text seems to be to promote eHealth services to healthcare professionals, to convince them of the usefulness of the new technology and that Vitaphone is the leading expert in this field. By describing the new technology as 'future-oriented' and 'innovative', the brochure text suggests that healthcare professionals should adopt Vitaphone products and services in order to remain 'modern'.[31] Compared to the traditional healthcare providers, telecare professionals are more frequently represented in the website and the brochure. This does not imply, however, that their perspectives are taken into account. The texts are restricted to describing their instrumental tasks. Any references to whether or how this new category of healthcare professionals may succeed in fulfilling its intermediary role between healthcare professionals and patients are absent from the text.

Although important concerns are thus not addressed, the promises articulated by Vitaphone are not restricted to positive expectations. In contrast to Philips, Vitaphone describes the problems they face in the implementation of the new technology. On the website, the company concludes:

> Despite all these benefits, which in part have been proven by international studies, telemedicine is only hesitantly winning recognition. One reason is that health insurances still abstain from financing the new technology and rewarding its application ... Although the technology is available, tele-cardiology is only slowly being implemented into normal everyday medical practice.[32]

The slow pace of implementation is, however, caused not only by resistance among health insurers. The rhetoric adopted in the brochure and on the website suggests that there are also disagreements with healthcare professionals. Both texts are carefully written to avoid the impression that telecare jeopardizes the autonomy of traditional healthcare professionals. On the website Vitaphone's services are described in terms of 'complementary services' and the telemedical centre is presented as 'the doctor's partner'[33] and not as an independent, separate organization.[34] The brochure texts emphasizes that

> Vitaphone's Medical Service Center ... provides effective support to doctors in the field. Their therapeutic autonomy and freedom are un-impinged.[35]

The brochure also tries to avoid the impression that telecare is a technology-driven development that will replace traditional healthcare professionals. Under the headline 'Main focus on people' the brochure text explains:

> However, despite all the enthusiasm for the potential of new technologies and the undeniably good reasons for using them, the main focus of attention has to be people and patients. eHealth should never become an end in itself. It provides support to doctors but it should not replace them or the face-to-face meetings in the surgery or the hospital.[36]

Overly optimistic expectations about cost reduction are tempered as well. The website describes the potential cost benefits of the new technology in terms of 'medium-term cost-reduction'.[37] Although Vitaphone thus articulates problems in realizing the promises of the new technology, they remain confident that e-health technologies will become successful in the near future. Referring again to Frost & Sullivan consultants, they conclude: 'In the next few years eHealth will make a great leap forward, especially in cardiology.'[38]

The ambulatory ECG recorder: Telemonitoring of heart-rhythm disturbances

Promises and scenario

Compared to the previous two telecare devices, the ambulatory ECG-recorder has the longest tradition in providing care at a distance. It was introduced into the Netherlands in 1995 by the Dutch firm Hartis. The company specializes in the detection of heart-rhythm abnormalities (cardiac arrhythmias) for general practitioners by telecare means. The main activities of the company are twofold. It provides general practitioners and home-care organizations with patient-activated ambulatory ECG recorders,[39] and it runs a telemedical centre where patients can have their recorded ECGs interpreted. The portable ECG-recorder is a device for registering, recording and transmitting ECGs developed to assist in the diagnosis of irregularities of the heart rhythm across distances. It consists of a round box that patients can clip to their waistbands, and three ECG electrodes that they have to attach to their bare chests (see Figure 3.4). When patients experience heart-rhythm problems, they have to activate the ambulatory ECG recorder manually to retain the current contents of the memory buffer, along with an additional post-event portion of the ECG signal. When patients have stored one or more ECG recordings (with a maximum of four), they have to contact

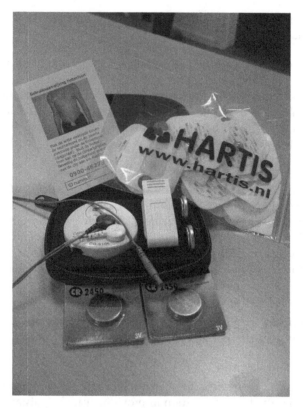

Figure 3.4   The ambulatory ECG-recorder

a telemedical centre, or Hartis Medical Center, as it is called. After a short anamnesis by the contacted physician, the patient has to send his or her recordings to the telemedical centre, where the ECGs emerge on a computer screen. In combination with the anamnesis the ECG is interpreted by the telephysician. This interpretation is directly passed on to the patient, and later, together with (parts of) the ECG, faxed to the patient's general practitioner who prescribed the device. If there is an emergency, the physician at the telemedical centre can call for an ambulance, and the general practitioner is informed immediately.

To attract the attention of potential users, Hartis runs a website that, in contrast to the websites of the other two firms, has adopted a rather modest, matter-of-fact-design that consists primarily of short texts.[40] Pictures of the device and a patient are included only on the home page and in the manual that can be downloaded from the website.

The major promise about the ambulatory ECG recorder is reflected in the name of the company: Hartis is an abbreviation of Hart (heart) and IS (Iedere Seconde = every second) to emphasize that in heart disorders every second counts to receive timely treatment that may save your life. On its website, the firm further specifies this expectation statement by articulating promises to patients, general practitioners and health insurers. The section 'Information for patients' promises patients that the use of the portable ECG recorder will create a 'reassured feeling', provide 'care in your own hand', 'reduce waiting lists' and 'avoid unnecessary referrals to the hospital'.[41] The section 'Information for general practitioners' also emphasizes that the use of the portable ECG-recorder will be beneficial to patients: the device will reduce patients' worries because they will be monitored for a longer period of time.

The first promise articulated in this section, however, directly addresses the interest of general practitioners by emphasizing that 'heart rhythm diagnostics will remain preserved for primary care' (Website Hartis, 2006). Although not explained further, this promise seems to refer to ongoing boundary work[42] about which profession should be responsible for the diagnosis of heart-rhythm disturbances: general practitioners (so-called first-line or primary care) or cardiologists (second-line or secondary care). Because most medical technological devices have been introduced in hospitals to be used by specialists, diagnostics has increasingly become the domain of healthcare professionals in secondary care. Consequently, the role of general practitioners is increasingly being restricted to referring patients to specialists in hospitals. Hartis promises general practitioners that the ambulatory ECG-recorder will help them to remain active in the field of diagnostics, particularly in diagnosing heart-rhythm disturbances based on ECGs. When patients visit their rooms with symptoms that suggest a heart-rhythm disorder, general practitioners are no longer dependent on cardiologists. They can make the diagnosis themselves and refer patients to the specialist care of cardiologists only when a serious abnormality is detected (interview Hollander, 2004). Hartis thus promises general practitioners that the use of the ambulatory ECG-recorder will help them to defend the authority and independence of their profession. Other promises to general practitioners include better registration of complaints (explaining that the ambulatory ECG-recorder will increase the chance of detecting a heart-rhythm disorder); more time for necessary care (referring to the time general practitioners will gain because they will receive fewer calls from patients worried about their hearts); and more efficient referral and shorter waiting lists for secondary care. The promise to health insurers also emphasizes more efficient referrals to hospitals. In addition, Hartis promises them that the use of the ambulatory ECG-recorder will introduce better service for their clients and decrease the use of 'more expansive secondary care'.[43]

In contrast to the promises articulated by Philips and Vitaphone, Hartis restricts its promises to reporting the state-of-the-art of the ambulatory ECG-recorder and its role in current healthcare. Their website does not claim that the telemonitoring device will contribute to directing the future of healthcare. This relatively modest strategy reflects the position of the company. In contrast to Philips, a newcomer in the field of telemedicine, and Vitaphone, a firm that partly adopts a direct-to-consumer strategy, Hartis has already established a position, though small, in Dutch healthcare. The firm has adopted a business model in which the ECG-recorder is not sold to patients but prescribed by general practitioners. Patients can receive the device at the general practitioner's office or a home-care organization where patients can collect the recorder and return it after use. Although the number of general practitioners actively involved in prescribing the device is still rather small, Hartis has succeeded in convincing several health insurers of the quality of their service, which have agreed to reimburse the costs of the device (interview Holwerda, 2004).[44]

The promises articulated in the website imply the following scenario. Patients will worry less about their heart problems because the ambulatory ECG-recorder will define whether or not they suffer from a serious heart disorder. They will be in control of care and can avoid waiting lists or unnecessary referrals to the hospital. General practitioners remain responsible for diagnosis of heart rhythm disturbances and save time for other patients. Finally, health insurers can reduce rising costs of secondary care by covering the telemonitoring device.

Actors and roles

The actors and roles defined in the scenario of the ambulatory ECG recorder are very straightforward. The design of the website, that is, the links on the home page where viewers can click to receive more information, distinguishes three groups of actors: patients, general practitioners, and healthcare insurers. The major role allocated to patients is that they have to make an appointment at a distribution centre to receive the ECG-recorder and instructions how to use it, and to record and send ECGs to the telemedical centre. After 30 days of use they have to return the device to the distribution centre. The roles allocated to general practitioners are formulated in similarly matter-of-fact language. They are expected to prescribe the ambulatory ECG-recorder to patients by downloading a specific form from the website and faxing the signed form to the telemedical centre. Consequently, they have to refer the patient to the nearest distribution centre. They also have to contact health insurers to charge the extra expenses of their work, which is set at a fixed amount of €25 per prescription. The roles allocated to health insurers are not framed in instructive terms but as an invitation:

> More and more health insurers become convinced of the role of the Hartis holterphone in heart-rhythm disturbances. We invite health insurers to become acquainted with our organization and working methods. Hartis is acknowledged as an adequate eHealth provision by Nitel [the Dutch governmental organization for the coordination of telecare initiatives].[45]

In contrast to the role of patients and general practitioners, the role of health insurers is obviously not taken for granted. Although some health insurers have agreed to reimburse the patients who use new technology (the website includes a list of six insurance companies), other insurers still have to be convinced that they should include the new technology in their services.

The text of the website also includes references to other groups of actors that are expected to play a role in realizing the scenario of the portable ECG-recorder: the healthcare staff at the Hartis Medical Centre (see Figure 3.5), described as 'the core of the service', and the employees at the distribution centres.

At the telemedical centre, 'specially trained physicians' are expected to evaluate the ECGs and 'take care of adequate follow-up', and to inform the treating physician about the ECGs, which includes a final report after the 30-day period of use.[46] The role of the healthcare staff at the distribution centre is mentioned only in two short sentences. They are expected to give instructions to patients and to make a test-ECG.

Compared to the other websites, the role the telecare device is expected to play receives rather limited attention on Hartis's website. The role allocated to the ambulatory ECG-recorder is simply to register ECGs. In addition to this instrumental role, the technology is expected to 'reduce the bottlenecks in the delivery of healthcare', a role which refers to Hartis's mission to 'reduce waiting lists, to decrease costs of secondary care, and to improve services for patients'.

Perspectives and silences

Like the other two scenarios, the scenario for the portable ECG-recorder prioritizes the perspective of some actors over the perspectives

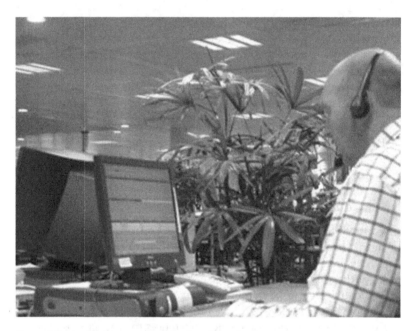

Figure 3.5   A physician at work in the telemedical centre

of others. In the website, Hartis explicitly addresses the concerns of patients, general practitioners, and health insurers. The section 'Information for patients' is clearly written from the perspective of patients. It informs patients about the advantages of using the telemonitoring device, emphasizing that they will remain in control while using the device. Under the headline 'Care in your own hands', the website informs patients that 'you monitor your heart-rhythm disturbances yourself', and 'you will decide yourself when you think it is necessary to record an ECG and ask for an evaluation'.[47] The text that informs patients about the indications for which the ambulatory ECG recorder can be prescribed also carefully adopts the perspective of patients by describing the symptoms of heart-rhythm disturbances in lay terms and avoiding complex medical explanations in expert language. The one-page manual that can be downloaded reflects a similar approach. The instructions are formulated in clear, short sentences written in lay terminology.

The information provided to general practitioners also adopts the perspective of this group of actors. As described above, the section

'Advantages' begins with the promise that 'heart-rhythm diagnostics will remain preserved for first-line care', thus promising general practitioners that the use of the new technology will support them in their struggle to preserve the authority of their profession in the field of cardiology care. The explanation of the other advantages also takes the concerns of general practitioners as a point of departure by emphasizing how the use of the telemonitoring device can assist them to spend more time on other necessary care. Although Hartis thus tries to take into account the perspectives and concerns of patients and general practitioners, the website merely addresses their instrumental actions. Concerns about how the use of the ambulatory ECG-recorder may affect the daily lives of patients, including the feeling of being at home, whether patients are willing to 'take care in their own hands', or whether some patients may not be willing or able to adopt this new role are not addressed. In a similar vein, the website takes it for granted that general practitioners are willing to prescribe the portable ECG-recorder to patients, and does not describe how the new technology will change their practices of care. However, the way in which Hartis defines its mission can be read as a reflection on possible resistance among general practitioners. As described above, the company articulates its contribution to healthcare in rather modest terms, labelling it as 'a complementary service' to heart-rhythm diagnosis.[48] Like Vitaphone, the company thus tries to avoid presenting its telemonitoring service as a technology that will replace current healthcare professionals; on the contrary, the new technology will assist general practitioners to become the prime actors in the diagnosis of heart-rhythm disturbances.

Finally, the website also briefly addresses the perspectives of health insurers by explaining how the use of the portable ECG-recorder will assist them 'to deliver better services to their clients, to reduce the costs of expensive second-line care, and to create more efficient collaboration between healthcare professionals'. In contrast to the other actors, the perspectives of healthcare staff at the telecare and distribution centres are, however, not addressed on the website. Although the scenario delegates a crucial role to physicians at the telemedical centre, the actual work and perspectives of this new category of healthcare professionals are not included in the text. Concerns about whether telecare staff will be able to provide care at a distance, and how this care interferes with or differs from face-to-face care, are not taken into account. Equally importantly, the website does not address concerns about how and whether healthcare professionals at the distribution centres will succeed in making patients familiar with the new technology and turning them into competent users of it.

Conclusions

Changing the order of who cares

Although the websites, press releases and brochures used to attract the attention of potential users of the three telecare devices analysed in this chapter articulate different promises, some promises are shared in the expectation statements for this new technology. Telecare devices for heart patients are expected to:

1 make healthcare more cost-effective and efficient by delegating care to telecare professionals and patients,
2 empower patients to take an active role in healthcare,
3 improve the quality of life,
4 improve the quality of care.

These promises paint a rather rosy future of the new technology.[49] By merely articulating the positive, enabling 'characteristics' of telecare devices, the expectation statements do not address the concerns, anxieties, or resistances involved in the changing landscape of care. The articulation of positive expectations at the expense of constraining aspects is thus not only part and parcel of the promises articulated during the early phase of technological innovation (Borup et al., 2006), but is also an important characteristic of the dynamics of promises when technologies are introduced into the market, not because constraints on the acceptance are not yet known, as is the case with promises in the early phase of technology, but because innovators are under pressure to make the introduction of new technologies a success because of the economic interests at stake. This may include the selling of telecare devices (Philips), or investment in telemedical centres (Achmea, Vitaphone and Hartis), or the economic position of the firm itself (Vitaphone and Hartis). In this context, websites are used as tools to create a positive and attractive image of the new technology.

Another related economic interest at stake in these promises is the contribution telecare technologies are expected to reduce the costs of healthcare. By portraying telecare technologies as tools to make healthcare more cost-effective and efficient, innovators contribute to the dominant discourse on the political economy of care by trying to convince policymakers of the relevance of the new technologies.

However, the emphasis on positive expectations cannot be ascribed only to economic concerns but is also related to the view of technology underlying these promises. In the websites and other information tools, telecare devices are (implicitly) considered as instrumental tools that facilitate healthcare. Consequently, they can simply add to or replace existing healthcare practices and traditions if potential users are convinced of the advantages of the new technology. As described in the previous chapter, the successful implementation of new technologies involves much more than simply introducing a device into its context of use (Berg and Mol, 1998; Webster, 2006; Lehoux, 2006). Drawing on the techno-geographical approach described earlier, we can conclude that the social and cultural changes involved in the redistribution of care over different places and actors, including changing responsibilities and interdependencies and the changing meanings of places where care takes place are largely absent in the promises articulated in relation to telecare devices. The only exceptions are the expectation statements about the heart mobile phone and, to a lesser extent, the ambulatory ECG-recorder, which refer to constraints on the diffusion of the new technology, indicating that there is resistance to the way in which telecare devices redistribute responsibilities among healthcare professionals.

The questions concerning the changing landscape of care that are silenced in the promises about these new technologies can be summarized as follows. First, we may wonder whether traditional healthcare professionals will be willing to delegate parts of the care they provide to telecare professionals and telemedical centres. Will they feel threatened because telecare may compete with, or even replace, their current practices of care? The next chapter addresses these questions by focusing on resistances among healthcare professionals to integrating these new technologies in their care practices. Second, it is important to understand whether and how the new telemedical centres will succeed in performing the 'crucial role' they are expected to play in realizing the scenarios of care at a distance. Who actually are these invisible telecare workers? What kind of new healthcare professionals are constituted in the telemedical centres? What constitutes the work practices of these intermediaries between patients, healthcare professionals, and technological devices? These questions are addressed in Chapter 5, which describes the emergence of telemedical centres and the work practices of telecare workers. Third, there is another category of healthcare professionals whose work remains largely invisible in the expectation statements, namely the staff involved in distributing the telecare devices and giving instructions to patients. The work of these healthcare providers is important in understanding how and whether patients will be able to adopt the active role in healthcare inscribed in the telecare devices, which are analysed in Chapter 7.

Creating new forms of care

Adopting a techno-geographical approach, we may expect that telecare technologies redefine not only the order of who cares but also where care takes place and what care will be provided. Although the promises on how telecare technologies will affect healthcare include far-reaching claims, that is, that telecare technologies will 'change the whole way healthcare is delivered' (Philips website, downloaded 25 November 2005), the actual consequences of these changes for the landscape of care are not taken into account. One of the major changes implied by the new technology, namely that physical contacts will be (partly) replaced by virtual contacts, is not addressed at all. What does it mean when care moves from physical to digital encounters? How important are places which enable physical contacts between doctors and patients? As with the term 'quality of life', 'quality of care' may not be an adequate term to capture the changes in care implied in telecare devices. As the promises indicate, quality of care can assume many different shapes, varying from preventing certain things from happening (e.g. admission to hospitals or anxiety about heart problems) to making things happen (e.g. disciplining patients to comply with a regime of medication and life style).

A discourse in terms of quality of care obscures what kinds of care are prioritized in telecare. What forms of care are constituted in the new telemedical centres? What gets lost and what is gained when doctor–patients encounters are mediated by telecare devices? Chapters 6 and 7 address these questions and show how places matter in healthcare.

Redefining patients and homes

As for healthcare professionals, the roles patients are expected to play to realize the scenarios for care at a distance are largely absent in the promises articulated on the websites and in other information tools. Although the promises of two telecare devices (the heart mobile phone and the ambulatory ECG-recorder) partly adopt the perspective of patients, the expectation statements are largely restricted to describing the instrumental tasks of patients and include a functionalistic perspective on how the technology will affect patients' lives. This particular way of representing patients is not restricted to promises on telecare devices for heart patients. Studies on telecare devices introduced to support the frail elderly to remain living at home have shown similar dynamics. Maggi Mort et al. (2009) have described how elderly patients are silenced in discourses on the design and governance of these telecare devices where patients are 'cast very much as 'passive players'. According to Mort, patients are represented as 'absent intermediaries' (Mort et al. 2009, 14, 21). In this respect we can conclude that promises on telecare technologies for heart patients adopt a less restricted view of patients because patients are not silenced or represented as passive but merely addressed in terms of their instrumental actions. However, major aspects of patients' roles and perspectives are nevertheless silenced in the expectation statements. For example, concerns whether patients are willing to receive care at a distance instead of physical contacts with their own family doctor or treating specialist are not addressed. By silencing other existing practices of care, websites enforce the use of telecare technologies as 'the only rational way of living with the disease' (Pols et al., 2008, p. 10). Also, websites do not pay attention to the anxieties patients may experience while using telecare devices, or how patients may acquire the knowledge and skills required to become competent users of the new technology. These questions become even more urgent because the new technology is not only meant to be used by younger patients but by a generation for whom digital devices are not part and parcel of daily life. Against this background it is even more surprising that the promises address patients as a homogeneous category without regard for the diversity among patients in terms of age, gender, and ethnicity. Will elderly women with hearing disabilities, for example, be able to master the use of ECG monitoring devices that operate via the phone? To what extent can telecare devices based only on Dutch be used by immigrants? Are younger patients willing to become disciplined by telecare devices? Although these concerns are important to fulfill the promise that telecare technologies will improve the quality of life of 'the patient', diversity among patients and processes of inclusion – and exclusion are not addressed in the expectation statements.

Last but not least, the promises are rather sketchy in describing how telecare devices will improve the quality of life of patients. Promises usually refer to a reduction of time spent in hospitals and waiting lists to receive specialist care, or how telecare devices will reduce the anxieties of patients. As other scholars have suggested, this approach to quality of life does not reflect on what sort of life is implicated in the use of telecare devices (Willems, 1995). What does the use of the new technology mean for the daily lives of heart patients? How does it affect their practices and experiences of being at home? Will the active involvement of patients in healthcare 'empower' patients by increasing their autonomy, or will it imply an increased dependency and medicalization? As we have seen, the expectation statements easily switch between very different approaches to making patients more active in healthcare, referring to notions of empowerment, patient compliance, and self-management. But are these approaches really the same, or are there conflicting norms and patient identities at stake?[50] What happens when patients 'take care in their own hands' (Hartis website) or become 'managers of their own health condition' (Motiva website)? Chapters 7 and 8 take up these issues and investigate whether and how patients are willing and able to perform the identity and actions ascribed to them, and how the use of telecare devices redefines patients' home and public spaces.

Promises, so what?

In the introduction to this Chapter, I began with the argument that technologies cannot exist without promises. My analysis illustrates that innovators are very active in articulating promises about telecare devices on their websites and other information tools. I showed how promises are largely restricted to articulating the instrumental tasks of actors considered important in realizing these promises and don't include broader changes in the landscape of care implicated in telecare technologies. We may wonder, however, whether this is a problem or not. We can downplay the importance of websites by suggesting that they are merely rhetorical tools used to sell a given technology. As described above, promises can be considered as important tools in attracting the interest of relevant audiences and mobilizing support to make the technology work. I suggest that there is more at stake than attracting audiences and mobilizing support. As Borup has already suggested, promises also function as instruments to create a specific identity of the technology. I want to extend this argument by suggesting that promises also play a role in imagining the identity of its users and the kind of care implicated in telecare technologies. By silencing the ways in which telecare technologies imply different kinds of patient, healthcare professional and care, the circulation of promises by websites may contribute to a situation in which patients, healthcare professionals, and, last but not least, policymakers are not prepared to anticipate and incorporate the changes implicated in telecare technologies into their practices and policies.

Like promises, silences are also not innocent. The following chapter addresses one of the silences in the promises of telecare devices. It describes how telecare devices disrupt the order of 'who cares' and analyses the resistances and negotiations involved in defending and redefining the boundaries between healthcare professionals.

4
Resistance and Boundary Work

> The fate of facts and machines is in later users' hands;
> their qualities are thus a consequence, not a cause, of
> a collective action.
>
> (Latour, 1987, p. 259)

Technical devices are intriguing objects. Advocates of new technologies often try to convince us that technologies will solve of society problems and improve our lives. This view of technology as problem-solver also dominates discourses on telecare technologies. As described in the previous chapter, telecare devices are expected to solve financial and labour problems in healthcare and simultaneously improve the quality of life and care. This discourse thus ascribes a kind of magic to technologies that may be very tempting to believe but will inevitably lead to disappointments. This also happened to the high hopes invested in telemedical technologies. Difficulties in the diffusion and acceptance of this new technology in the last decade indicate that the promises articulated by the innovative firms are not as readily fulfilled as expected. Whereas Vitaphone and Hartis found fewer patients willing to use their telecare devices,[1] Philips met with resistance from doctors reluctant to collaborate with the new category of telecare professionals when they introduced their heart-failure telemonitoring system in Europe.[2] Actors who are supposed to play an important role in realizing the promises of the new technology thus appear unwilling to step forward to fulfil the roles attributed to them in the expectation statements. Obviously, patients and healthcare professionals are not (yet?) convinced that the new technology will solve problems and improve healthcare. Resistance is not restricted to the three telemonitoring devices analysed in this book; other telecare technologies are also meeting with resistance. Despite the many pilot studies and clinical trials conducted to develop and implement the new technology in the US and Europe, telecare technologies have not yet developed into regular care practices in any systematic manner (Mair et al., 2004; May et al., 2004; Mattke, 2011). To understand this resistance, it is important to abandon the view of technology as a problem-solver. Adopting a techno-geographical approach to technology, we may expect telecare technologies to redistribute responsibilities and create interdependencies between people, places, and technological devices. In this process, the identities of technical objects and humans are also (re)configured. As described in the previous chapter, telecare technologies imply that the healthcare traditionally provided by cardiologists and general practitioners will be delegated partly to patients and the new category of telecare workers, thus reconfiguring their responsibilities, agency, and identities. The introduction of telecare technologies thus implies changes in long-standing traditions and practices of care and challenges to professional and patient identities. It seems likely that these changes in the landscape of care would meet with resistance.

In this chapter I investigate this resistance and show how the introduction of telecare devices disturbed the order of care in a very specific way, by challenging the professional autonomy and authority of medical professionals. Studies of the relationships between medical technologies and healthcare professionals have shown how the introduction of new technologies usually plays an important role in establishing, maintaining, or extending the expertise and authority of medical professionals (Lehoux, 2006 p. 63). The introduction of imaging technologies, for example, has contributed to the status of radiology as a medical specialty since World War I (Blume, 1992). Technologies can thus play a role in establishing and maintaining the boundaries of a professional group's authority over who is allowed to perform certain tasks (Abbott, 1988; Freidson, 1975). Telecare technologies, however, do not fit into this picture. In contrast to other medical technologies, telecare technologies contest rather than sustain professional boundaries. Drawing on Abbot's seminal work on how the development of expert professions can be understood in terms of inter-professional competitions, I analyse how boundary work between healthcare professionals has shaped the implementation of telecare technologies. I use the concept of boundary work[3] to refer to the work involved in maintaining healthcare professionals' authority over their qualifications (Abbott, 1988). Whereas Abbott has shown how technologies can lead to interprofessional contests, I extend his argument by showing the reciprocal interrelations between technologies and the maintenance of professional autonomy: telecare technologies both initiate and are shaped by boundary work among healthcare professionals.

My account of resistance and boundary work performed during the introduction and use of telecare technologies is based on an analysis of the websites of the producers of telecare devices and interviews with relevant actors involved in the implementation and use of telecare technologies in Germany and the Netherlands. I focus on resistance related to two of the three telecare devices for heart patients discussed in this book: the heart mobile phone that assists patients at risk of heart attacks and the telecare system for heart-failure patients.[4] In this chapter I show how the boundary work of traditional healthcare professionals involved a defence not only of their professional authority to keep specific aspects of care in their own hands, but also defined the boundaries of the new profession of telecare workers. Most importantly, these contestations about who cares not only shaped the boundaries of medical professions; they also redefined the identity of users of the technology and established norms for what should be considered good care. First, I describe how the boundary work of general practitioners redefined the identity of the heart mobile phone and its intended users. Then, I analyse how healthcare professions contested and defined the boundaries of the new professions of telecare workers, a process that included the redesign of the software of the heart-failure telemonitoring system.

Redefining the identity of users and devices

Constituting patients as clients

When the heart mobile phone was introduced in Germany in 1999, it was a novelty. As described in Chapter 2, the so-called Herz Handy or Cardiophone was the first mobile phone capable of recording, storing, and transmitting ECGs. However, the new telecare device was a novelty not only in terms of its technical content: the heart mobile phone was among the first technologies designed to reconfigure the user of ECG-recording devices. As the ambulatory ECG-recorder, the heart mobile phone configured users as patients rather than healthcare professionals. Ever since the introduction of the first ECG-recording technologies in the early 1910s, the recording of ECGs had been the exclusive domain of cardiologists, and sometimes general practitioners. The introduction of telecare devices for making and sending ECGs meant that for the first time in history patients could make ECGs themselves. Another technological innovation facilitated the intended shift in primary users of telecare ECG devices: Vitaphone advertised the Cardiophone on its website, where patients could order the new technology directly. The choice of this direct-to-consumer marketing and selling, instead of a sales strategy based on prescription by cardiologists or general practitioners, was made because of the long period involved in formal procedures for the approval of medical technologies. In Germany, medical technological devices are approved for inclusion in the so-called prescription list of the Ministry of Health and insurance companies only after a 3–5-year period of studies that show the benefits of the new technology (Interview Sack, 2004).

Following a change in the Medical Product Law in 2002, producers of medical technologies were allowed to advertise their products directly to the consumer market. This change in the German regulatory regime enabled Vitaphone to sell the heart mobile phone directly to patients, which promised to be faster and to guarantee bigger sales than the route via doctors' prescriptions (Interview Quinger, 2004).

One major consequence of this choice is that patients are constituted as clients, or 'Kunden' as users of the Cardiophone are called in the software system of the telemedical centre. The heart mobile phone was thus related to a third novelty. In contrast to the US, where direct-to-consumer marketing is part and parcel of the healthcare system, Germany and other European countries have tried to introduce this approach only gradually in the past decade. The heart mobile phone fitted into this new, neo-liberal approach to healthcare delivery. However, this move towards a new political economy of healthcare turned out to be one bridge too far. In contrast to the promises and expectations articulated by the innovators, the Cardiophone did not reach high sales numbers. First, patients did not order a heart mobile phone via Vitaphone's website very frequently (Interview Quinger, 2004). Particularly patients at risk of heart attacks, described on Vitaphone's website as one of the target groups of the heart mobile phone, were not interested in the new technology at all (Interview Sack, 2004). But also patients who had experienced a heart attack already were not inclined to buy a heart mobile phone. Although patients may have acknowledged the potential benefits of the technology, they did not want to pay for the device themselves. This reluctance can be understood in the context of the German health-insurance system, where costs of diagnoses and medical therapy are usually reimbursed by health-insurance companies. According to Matthias Quinger, director of Vitaphone, the health-insurance system has created an attitude among patients that he described as a 'Voll-Kasko Mentalitat' (an all-risk assurance attitude): patients are simply not used to paying for medical services themselves. Reflecting on their strategy to sell directly to patients, Quinger concluded that 'the firm has been misled by the promising prospects of the consumer market' (Interview Quinger, 2005).

At first sight, the reluctance of patients to buy a heart mobile phone can be considered as voting with their feet: patients are not purchasing the new technology because they see only cost-related disadvantages. However, patients' resistance cannot be ascribed only to individual choices, but should also be understood in the context of the changes in the landscape of care inscribed in the heart mobile phone. Or, as the inventor of the cardiophone described his experiences:

> There are cardiologists who are rather sceptic[al] and think they themselves have to decide when an ECG is recorded and not the patients.
>
> (Interview Sack, 2004)

By configuring patients instead of healthcare professionals as primary users, the heart mobile phone disturbed the order of care in which the responsibility for using and prescribing medical devices had been delegated to healthcare professionals. The heart mobile phone drastically challenged this central position of cardiologists and general practitioners as gatekeepers in healthcare.[5] The reluctance of patients should therefore also be understood in terms of the boundary work of healthcare professionals. Or as Vitaphone's director described his experiences with the implementation of the heart mobile phone:

> We thought people would like the idea of a mobile phone with the addition to check the heart. We thought it would make them feel good, and health and lifestyle is the trend nowadays, but the physicians said no.
>
> (Interview Quinger, 2004)

Boundary work and redesign

The company thus experienced fierce resistance from medical professionals. Whereas cardiologists were not convinced of the benefits of telemedical technologies (Interview Sack, 2004), general practitioners considered the new technology as a threat to their profession. This threat was of two kinds. On the one hand, the heart mobile phone intervened into the physician's professional autonomy because it was directly sold to patients, thus bypassing physicians as gatekeepers in the prescription of devices to register ECGs. To quote Quinger again:

> We want to bring the pressure via the customer to the healthcare system. That people tell their physician that they need it. That they have seen it on TV, or in the newspaper, and that they want it. But physicians do not want this. They are angry because patients go away.
>
> (Interview Quinger, 2004)

On the other hand, the telecare device also challenged the authority of physicians because parts of their diagnostic tasks were transferred to Vitaphone' telemedical centre:

> The biggest sector is the consumer sector. But we do not come to the consumer if the physicians say no. Our first step in the market is to go to the pharmacies. People there see our product and want to buy it, but first they ask the physician and then the physician says: 'No, you do not need this. You can come to my office and we will make an ECG and see what has happened.' Therefore we grow so slowly, that we need very much money to survive this problem. The problem with physicians is that they think that we take over their patients. They see us as competitors.
>
> (Interview Quinger, 2004)

Physicians thus did not consider the heart mobile phone as a tool to improve care for heart patients but as a technology that would take away their patients. Physicians perceived the telemedical centre as a rival for the care provided to heart patients; they were not at all willing to delegate part of this care to the new profession of telecare workers.

To find new clients for its products and to avoid a situation in which the heart mobile phone would further increase inter-professional competition between physicians and telecare professionals, Vitaphone decided to redesign the product. The company had failed to make the heart mobile phone into a commodity for the consumer market, so it redesigned the Cardiophone in such a way that it would become a potential useful technology for general practitioners and cardiologists by enabling the user to see the ECG. In discussions with Vitaphone, physicians had told the firm that the heart mobile phone could be useful for their practices if they would redesign it with the ECG visible on the screen. While demonstrating the new heart mobile phone to me, Quinger explained:

> No, it's not for the patient. A normal patient doesn't have the knowledge to understand an ECG. It is for physicians. They can take the phone with them in their emergency box.
>
> (Interview Quinger, 2004)

This redesign added not only a screen to display ECGs but also involved a change from a so-called one-channel to a three-channel ECG-recording system. Owing to criticism from cardiologists and general practitioners that a one-channel (or one-lead) ECG was not good enough to diagnose a patient's condition, Vitaphone decided to include the three-channel ECG-system in the Cardiophone because it provided more detailed ECG representations (Interview Sack, 2004). In reaction to the boundary work of general practitioners and cardiologists, the heart mobile phone was redesigned from a technology that could be used by patients in emergencies into a device that could be used by healthcare professionals to diagnose patients during (emergency) visits at patients' homes or consulting hours at the doctor's rooms. In this new constellation, patients will use the heart mobile phone only when a cardiologist or general practitioner considers it important to receive regular ECGs from patients discharged from hospital who use the device for short period of time, usually a week (Interview Sack, 2004).

This redefinition of the identity of the primary user and the technology itself is clearly reflected in the update of the website Vitaphone introduced in 2006. The new version of the website is no longer organized around the various telemedical devices of the company. Instead it presents disease categories for which the devices can be used as diagnostic or monitoring tools, namely 'cardiac arrythmias, heart failure, hypertension, and diabetes mellitus', and it shows a picture of a doctor wearing a stethoscope on the home page.[6] The use of medical, Latin terminology for diseases shows a shift in primary target group from patients to healthcare professionals. In contrast to the version of the website analysed in the previous chapter, information on the heart mobile phone is much more hidden. Whereas the 2004 version showed the heart mobile phone directly on the home page, information on this device can now be found only by navigating the web pages. The heart mobile phone is included as one of the three telemedical devices in the webpage about the Vitaphone Service

Centre under the label 'Information for patients'. By clicking this label, the viewer will find a short explanation of the telemedical centre and descriptions of three mobile phones, with the heart mobile phone mentioned as the third device. By clicking on 'Technical Details', the viewer can download a brochure on the Herz Handy. The brochure is still the same as the version included in the first website. As we have seen in the previous chapter, the brochure text is clearly targeted to healthcare professionals as intended users of the telemedical products and services of Vitaphone. The new version of the website thus contains much less information for patients than the original website. This change in audience does concern not only the way in which the technologies are presented but also the manner in which heart diseases are described. The use of medical classifications of disorders as the main organizing principle of the website and the deletion of the webpage 'All about the heart', a page explaining the functioning and disorders of the heart in high-school textbook language, clearly show how Vitaphone reconfigured the users of the heart mobile phone as healthcare professionals and no longer as patients. The only page targeted at patients is the section Frequently Asked Questions that is still included in the website.

The redesign of the heart mobile phone thus resulted in a radically different position of the new technology in the changing landscape care. Whereas the Cardiophone was originally designed as a technology meant to be used by patients to gain access to medical care in emergency situations, the boundary work of general practitioners converted the new technology into a diagnostic tool for general practitioners. Consequently, the heart mobile phone became embedded in healthcare in a way similar to the other ECG-recording devices of Vitaphone. Like the ECG-cards, electronic cards that patients can use to register and store ECGs subsequently sent via mobile phone or land phone to the attending physician, the heart mobile phone became a technology for which healthcare professionals remained the gatekeepers and primary users. Nevertheless, cardiologists and general practitioners seem to prefer to use ECG-cards rather than the Cardiophone because the ECGs are directly forwarded by e-mail to their office (Interview Quinger, 2004; Interview Sack, 2004). This preference implies a major loss in the original potential of the telecare technologies for heart patients as articulated in the promises on the first website. In contrast to the heart mobile phone, ECG-cards are only a diagnostic tool; they do not include a GPS function and thus cannot be used to detect the position of the patient in need of emergency care.

Contesting and taming a new healthcare profession

Clinical trials as implementation strategy

Medical devices have a relatively free life. Compared to the introduction of new drugs or other medical therapies, there are no extensive rules for approval and admission to the market. Whereas for some 30 years pharmaceuticals have been subjected to international regulations based on internationally approved research protocols and methods, the regulation of medical technologies, including standards and protocols for clinical studies, is still in its infancy (Altenstetter, 2003, p. 114). In Europe as well as the US, the responsibility for testing the efficacy and safety of medical devices is largely left to producers of new technologies (Santen, 2008). This does not mean that the introduction of new medical devices does not involve tests or clinical studies. The field of telemedical technologies, for example, shows an abundance of pilot studies, or sometimes clinical trials, often financed by national governments or health insurers, at least in Europe. The role of governmental agencies is, however, different from their role in drug testing: they function not as inspectors or legal regulators, but as facilitators or advocates of the new technology.

The difference in regulatory regime between drugs and medical devices has major consequences for the kinds of clinical trial that are conducted for telecare technologies. First, the content of clinical studies is much more open to what producers consider relevant to include in the studies. Most clinical studies of telemedical technologies, including the clinical trials of telecare technologies for heart patients, include topics such as technical feasibility, cost-effectiveness, and quality of life, issues often articulated in the promises of the new technology as well. Second, producers can decide to introduce the new technology into the market even when clinical studies do not deliver the expected outcomes, as in the clinical studies on the heart-failure telemonitoring system. Although the clinical trial conducted in the Netherlands did not provide any significant data to confirm cost-effectiveness or improved quality of life, Philips decided to introduce the new technology in the European market (Interview Balk, 2007; interview Leussen, 2007).[7]

We thus may wonder why firms bother to conduct clinical trials if they are not required by law and the results do not influence their decisions. The case of the telecare system for heart-failure patients indicates a role for clinical trials beyond finding governmental approval or testing clinical and other parameters. Clinical trials can be used as strategic instruments to convince others of the benefits of the new technology and to create alliances with actors required to making the technology work. My argument is that clinical trials can also be understood as implementation instruments: they can be used as tools to enrol relevant actors and to anticipate and influence potential resistance to the new technology. The organization of clinical studies is important because it involves the creation of relationships with one of the major groups of actors required to build networks: clinicians. The enrolment of clinicians as so-called principal investigators facilitates a process in which important gatekeepers in healthcare become involved in the testing and implementation of the new technology. Clinicians are extremely relevant for innovations in healthcare, not only because they guard the boundaries of what changes in healthcare are acceptable for their professions but also because they negotiate exchanges between the world of technology and the world of medicine. Medical experts involved in clinical studies will disseminate the results of trials among their colleagues by writing articles for publication in medical journals and presenting papers at academic conferences. In this way, they will spread the news about the new technology in the medical world.

The innovators involved in the introduction of the telecare system for heart-failure patients clearly tried to use clinicians' capacity as gatekeepers. As the innovation manager of Achmea, the health insurer, that financed the clinical trial and operated the telemedical centre, described their strategy:

> When you want to innovate you'll have to find white ravens first: people who are interested in innovations because of their ideology or status and not because of financial profits ... This is very important for innovations, otherwise you will enter existing systems and meet resistance. By using my informal network I look for people described by their colleagues as innovative.
>
> (Interview Leussen, 2007)

The search for 'white ravens' was, however, not an easy job. Many cardiologists who were invited to participate in the clinical study Achmea and Philips organized in the Netherlands to introduce the new technology in the European market refused to take part in the trial. Cardiologists were not inclined to participate because of their busy work schedule, the low fee they received for their contributions, or because they considered the new technology as a competitor to their own well-functioning heart-failure polyclinic (Interview Leussen, 2007; interview Helm and Boutkan, 2006; interview Balk, 2005). Another major source of resistance was that cardiologists did not like the idea that the telemedical centre was owned and run by a health-insurance company. They did not want any interference by health insurers who would have access to information about their patients. Although health insurers would eventually become the major financiers of the whole telecare system [hospitals did not want to pay for the new technology because they considered telecare as care provided outside the hospital], some cardiologists nevertheless refused to participate in the clinical trial because health insurers should not have control over their patients (Interview Balk, 2005; Interview Leussen, 2007; interview Helm and Boutkan, 2006; interview Weijde, 2006).

The innovators encountered resistance not only from medical professionals. Clinicians who agreed to participate in the clinical study did not stick to their role of 'white ravens'. During the clinical testing of the new technology, clinicians became aware of (in their view), the negative consequences of the technology for their profession and the care they provided to heart-failure patients. Consequently, the white ravens turned into black ravens, to paraphrase Achmea's metaphor: they began to contest one of the central constitutive elements of the new technology: the telemedical centre and the profession of telecare workers.

Boundary work: Control over patients

The resistance to the telemedical centre and its staff that emerged during the clinical testing of the heart-failure telemonitoring system is not very surprising. The history of medicine gives ample examples of how the entry of a new medical profession has been heavily criticized and contested by the already established professions (Freidson, 1975). Some of the resistance to the healthcare professionals participating in the clinical trials can indeed be understood as straightforward boundary work: the introduction of a new infrastructure and a new category of healthcare workers was considered a potential threat to the existing practices of healthcare for heart-failure patients. The introduction of the heart-failure telemonitoring system did not simply fill in a blank spot in healthcare; it provided an alternative way to monitor heart-failure patients.

Since the mid-1990s, major hospitals in the Netherlands have established special outpatients' departments, known as heart-failure polyclinics, staffed by the newly established nursing specialty of heart-failure nurses. Consequently, care traditionally given by cardiologists has been partly delegated to this new category of nurses. Given the rather recent introduction of heart-failure polyclinics, it can easily be imagined that the introduction of the heart-failure telemonitoring system was considered as a potential competitor. One of the heart-failure nurses participating in the clinical study expressed this so aptly: 'Everyone is drawing on the patient' (Interview heart-failure nurse A,[8] October 2006). Participating cardiologists considered it important that the new technology would not break up their heart-failure polyclinics (Interview Balk, 2005).

For heart-failure nurses, the newcomer was even more disturbing because telecare workers threatened the very existence of their profession. Both telecare by telenurses and physical monitoring by heart-failure nurses were developed to bridge the gap between the growing demand for care of chronic heart-failure patients because of an ageing population and the limited number of healthcare professionals and available financial resources. However, the healthcare services have adopted two different approaches to resolving the tension between demand and resources. Heart-failure polyclinics represent a strategy that aims to reduce costs by delegating tasks and responsibilities from cardiologists to less expensive specialized nurses. Telecare technologies for heart-failure patients go one step further by delegating care to a new healthcare infrastructure (the telemedical centre), a new category of healthcare staff (telecare workers), and, last but not least, new technological devices. Although these two different strategies – replacing people by people or replacing people partly by technologies – are not necessarily mutually exclusive, heart-failure nurses were nevertheless afraid that telecare workers would take over their work, or at least some of their patients (Interview Leussen, 2007; interview Borst, 2006; interview Helm and Boutkan, 2006).

The experiences of heart-failure nurses participating in the clinical study reduced some of these fears but simultaneously reinforced other worries. On the one hand, they saw that telecare professionals would not take over their job completely because physical contact with patients remained the responsibility of the heart-failure nurse. During the clinical trial patients were not only monitored by the telemedical system but also kept their appointments with the heart-failure polyclinic. What would happen after the trial was not clear. Managers of Achmea tried to reassure heart failure nurses that they would not lose their patients to the telemedical centre when the telecare system was implemented into healthcare. They argued that the new technology would result in a sorting of patients whereby those in need of more intensive care – so-called difficult patients - would visit the heart-failure polyclinic and other patients would be monitored by telecare workers

(Interview Helm and Boutkan, 2006). On the other hand, participation in the clinical study strengthened the heart-failure nurses' resistance to telecare workers because the collaboration with their new colleagues indicated tensions between the two professions. Promises that the telecare system would support the care provided by heart-failure nurses and cardiologists were not easy to realize. These tensions included conflicts about norms of care, which I will discuss in the next section, and control over the organization of work.

With respect to the organization of work, heart-failure nurses were annoyed by the fact that telecare workers tried to set the pace of their work. They received mail messages at moments that did not fit their work schedule from telenurses who told them what they should do and what they should not forget in their contacts with patients (Interviews heart-failure nurses A and C, 2006). These tensions were caused by the script of the heart-failure system, which received data from patients in the morning, and the division of tasks by which telecare staff was not allowed to change medications. Consequently, they were obliged to contact the heart-failure polyclinic when patients' data indicated the need for an intervention in medication. The coordination work and the use of the telemonitoring system also turned out to be rather time-consuming. Instead of a reduction in work, heart-failure nurses experienced an increase in their workload. Initially this was not considered a huge problem because the extra work was partly temporary: heart-failure nurses had to invest time in becoming familiar with retrieving and reading e-mail messages and learning to make decisions based on the information provided by the telenurses (Interview heart-failure nurse B, 2006). During the trial, heart-failure nurses became more negative about the extra work and began to perceive the telemedical centre as an unnecessary, extra intermediary between the patients and themselves. They appreciated the heart-failure telemonitoring system but wanted to receive patients' data on their own computer screens in the policlinic and not via the 'detour' of the telemedical centre (Interviews heart-failure nurse A, 2007 and nurse B, 2006). Or as one of the heart-failure nurses involved in the clinical trial and the training of the telenurses explained:

> I experienced the telemedical centre as negative. This was not because of the people working there but because it is an extra link between us and the patient. When a patient gains weight, the telenurse will see it on her screen. She will call the patient and send an e-mail to me to inform me about what happened. Then I have to call the patient

again, because I do not trust information from a second source. Then the patient tells me the story again and I will change medication, which I will have to report in the system. Therefore it takes half an hour you'll have to spend on the patient. If I could see the data on my own screen and could change medication directly it would not take so much time. I do not want anything between the patient and me. I want to do it myself.

(Interview heart-failure nurse A, 2007)

Heart-failure nurses thus did not want to delegate part of their work to telenurses, but want to keep care in their own hands.

Like heart-failure nurses, cardiologists participating in the clinical study, including the principal investigator, considered the telemedical centre as a time-consuming, unnecessary detour:

I am not critical of how the telemedical centre works. Nothing went wrong because of the telemedical centre. But it simply takes too much unnecessary time. You try to save time by these systems, but it only consumes time. Of course I want to do something extra, but it should become profitable elsewhere. Now it takes more time without giving any advantages.

(Interview Balk, 2007)

The irony is that some of the problems that emerged during the trial, that is, that the route via the telemedical centre was too time-consuming, were a result of boundary work before the clinical study began. In the preparatory meetings between the cardiologist who acted as principal investigator of the trial and the innovators it was agreed that telecare professionals would not be allowed to treat patients themselves – the responsibility for medical care would remain in the hands of the treating cardiologists and heart-failure nurses. The cardiologist would maintain his/her final responsibility for heart-failure patients, also in juridical terms (Interview Balk, 2007; interview Helm and Boutkan, 2006). Potential conflicts concerning who was entitled to provide medical care to patients were thus pre-empted by demarcating the qualifications and responsibilities that would be solely in the hands of cardiologists and heart-failure nurses. Tasks and responsibilities delegated to the new profession of telecare workers remained restricted to advice and assistance work rather than intervention. Telecare workers were allowed only to monitor and counsel patients; all medical intervention tasks were explicitly excluded from their qualifications (Interview Weijde, 2006).

Consequently, the new profession received a subordinate position in healthcare in which they were allowed to do only certain tasks under the control of the dominant profession of cardiology. The telecare profession became constituted as a facilitating rather than a treating profession. Before the clinical trial began, cardiologists and heart-failure nurses thus succeeded in drawing monopolizing boundaries around tasks and responsibilities they considered as their own jurisdictional work domain, a process that has happened many times before when new groups have tried to enter the world of medicine (Larson, 1979).

Conflicting norms of care

Heart-failure nurses and cardiologists participating in the clinical study of the telecare system thus wanted to keep care in their own hands. Their fierce boundary work can, however, be ascribed not only to protecting their workload and the autonomy or their profession but also to conflicting norms of care. One of the norms of care underlying their resistance towards the telemedical centre was related to the relationship between doctor and patient: in order to provide good care to heart-failure patients, you have to know the patient. In their view, you cannot provide proper care to heart-failure patients if you have not seen the patient before. Knowing and seeing patients is thus considered as important in caring for heart-failure patients, a practice I will analyse in more detail in Chapter 7. Because telecare professionals never meet the patient in person, they were not considered qualified to give medical treatment to heart-failure patients. Or, as one of the participating cardiologists explained:

> I did not like that call centre. On paper it seemed a nice idea. When you talk to people working there they know many things, but it does not work. I prefer heart-failure nurses who know the patients: they are close to them, know their language and speak with their accent. Patients can now only contact a call centre where they have to talk about their problem with a stranger.
>
> (Interview Leenders, 2007)

Knowing the patient was considered important not only because of social contacts with patients but also because telecare workers could make different assessments of the patients' problems:

> The telemedical centre may lead to mistakes because they cannot make the right assessment. People who know patients personally

very well may make another assessment of the problem than people
who only have contact by phone and this technical link [the telecare
system; N.O.].

(Interview Balk, 2005)

Although serious mistakes did not happen during the trial (Interview
Balk, 2005) and risks were reduced because of the agreement that telecare
staff would not do any medical interventions, there were tensions and
conflicts between heart-failure nurses and telecare workers that reveal
other (implicit) norms of care. One of the recurring conflicts included
decisions about medication. Although telecare professionals were not
allowed to change medication, the telecare system provided them with
information on changes in the patient's condition that could possibly
be solved by changing the dose of the prescribed drugs. When patients
gain weight, which suggests a retention of fluid near the lungs, one of
the symptoms of heart-failure, the telecare staff receive a signal, 'a flag',
on their computer screen to inform them that the patient has exceeded
the standards set for their weight. When telenurses subsequently
phoned or e-mailed the heart-failure polyclinic, the heart-failure nurses
sometimes did not want to change medication because they thought
it was too early to intervene, or that the deviation from the standards
was not serious enough to warrant a change of medication (Interview
heart-failure nurse A, 2006). On other occasions, telenurses asked heart-
failure nurses to change the standards set for weight because patients
frequently exceeded them and telehealthcare workers received too
many 'flags' from the system. Or as a telephysician explained:

Sometimes patients do not keep [to] their diet and gain weight, so we
receive flags very frequently. If patients do not change their behaviour we call the polyclinic to ask them to readjust the flag. Otherwise
you go nuts when you see the flag lightning on your screen every
day. Then we discuss a change in standards.

(Interview Borst, 2006)

Heart-failure nurses were sometimes not inclined to change the values
because in their view the patient should have been putting more effort
into adherence to the weight restrictions. They considered frequent
reminders as important information for patients because this encouraged them to keep trying to reduce their weight (Interview heart-failure
nurse B, 2006). The script of the telecare system thus triggered conflicts
between the ways in which heart-failure nurses wanted to provide care,

on the one hand, and the frustrations of telecare staff, on the other. Another norm of care scripted in the telecare system that violated the way in which heart-failure nurses and cardiologists were used to providing care was that it reduced the responsibility of patients to take care of themselves. Frequent phone calls of telecare staff were considered as too coercive to stimulate patients to adhere to their medication and lifestyle regime (Interview heart-failure nurse A, 2006; interview Burgh, 2007).

Finally, there were tensions between heart-failure nurses and telecare staff about the proper way to approach patients. According to heart-failure nurses, knowing patients personally is very important, particularly in the case of conveying messages that patients may not like, such as requests to change lifestyle. Patients sometimes complained to heart-failure nurses about the way they were approached by telecare professionals (Interview heart-failure nurse A, 2007). A cardiologist considered the way in which telenurses communicated with patients as negative for patients' condition because their approach increased patients' worries unnecessarily (Interview Leenders, 2007).

Bypassing the telemedical centre

Although cardiologists, heart-failure nurses, and telecare professionals collaborated with each other for more than a year, the clinical trial did not result in a peaceful settlement of inter-professional competition. Eventually, the cardiologists decided that they wanted to use the telecare technology only if the data collected from patients were sent directly to the heart-failure polyclinic. In their view, the telemedical centre did not provide any 'additional value' but only disturbed their work practices and threatened their norms of care (Interview Balk, 2007; interview Leenders, 2007; interview Burgh, 2007; interview heart-failure nurse A, 2007). Cardiologists wanted to keep care in their own hands, even more so because the telemedical centre operated only during office hours and week days (Interview Balk, 2005; interview Schroeder, 2008). The boundary work thus resulted in the bypassing of the telemedical centre and its staff. In meetings between the innovators and the principal investigator, it was agreed that hospitals that wanted to use the telecare system after the clinical study was completed were not obliged to 'use' the telemedical centre as well. Although the healthcare insurer tried to reach an agreement in which the telecare system would be offered as a one-package deal consisting of the telecare system and the telemedical centre that would receive a quality mark 'approved by cardiologists', the principal investigator, acting on behalf of the other cardiologists, explicitly rejected this proposal (Interview Balk, 2007).

After the trial, the first Dutch hospital to use the telecare system for a test period of a year also decided to bypass the telemedical centre. Like the cardiologists participating in the clinical study, the leading cardiologists there did not want to delegate part of the care they provided to heart-failure patients to healthcare professionals who did not know their patients. Another important reason was that the hospital had a well-functioning heart-failure polyclinic. The hospital, located in Amsterdam, was nevertheless interested in the telecare system because they expected that heart-failure nurses would not be able to maintain quality of care in the future because of the expected increase in heart-failure patients (Interview Schroeder and Beurs, 2008). They therefore decided to use the telecare system but demanded that patients' data be sent directly to their heart-failure polyclinic.

This turn from telehealth-care staff to heart-failure nurses as users of the telecare system had consequences not only for the telemedical centre but also for the telecare technology itself. When heart-failure nurses began to use the system, they became annoyed because the software programme was clearly not designed to be used by qualified nurses with expertise in caring for heart-failure patients. In their view, the system was designed according to the logic of computer experts and not adjusted to practices of care in the heart-failure polyclinic. Although the telecare system had received an award in the US because it was 'user-friendly' for patients, for heart-failure nurses the system was a 'nightmare'. They experienced the system as very inconvenient and time-consuming to use: the script of the software programme required that heart-failure nurses follow very extensive menus with questions they considered irrelevant or impractical in providing care to patients. Heart-failure nurses could not understand the computer terms used in the programme and complained that the system was not based on disease categories or diagnostic procedures used in the practice of caring for heart-failure patients (Interview Schroeder and Beurs, 2008).

This mismatch between design and use context meant that heart-failure nurses became enrolled in a redesign of the software programme for the telecare system, which involved weekly meetings with representatives of Philips to discuss the changes required to attune the software programme to the new group of users. Heart-failure nurses and cardiologists thus became co-designers of the telecare technology. After several months, they decided to stop doing this because the system had been improved enough to be used in the heart-failure polyclinic and the involvement in the redesign was too time-consuming. They had expected a system that would function very well, but instead they had to put quite some time into making the system useful to their work. Or, as the leading cardiologist told Philips:

> When I buy a car I can use it immediately. With the telecare system we first have to invest much time in it to be able to use it, work for which we do not receive anything at all.
>
> (Interview Schroeder, 2008)

Although the telecare system became embedded in the practice of the heart-failure polyclinic, the new situation challenged one of the promises of the new technology, namely, that it would make healthcare more cost-effective and labour efficient. By bypassing the telemedical centres, the workload of the heart-failure polyclinic increased rather than decreased. Heart-failure nurses received three times as many phone calls from patients because of the telecare system. Consequently, the hospital in Amsterdam realized that they could not implement the system in this way because they did not have enough staff to operate the telecare system, particularly if the number of patients were to increase. Their solution was to organize a local centre for all the hospitals in Amsterdam using the telecare system that could then be operated by heart-failure nurses in all the hospitals on a rotational basis (Interview Schroeder, 2008). In this way, cardiologists would be able to keep care in their own hands.

Conclusions

Reflecting on my analysis of the resistance of healthcare professionals to the implementation of telecare systems for heart patients, I can conclude that the boundary work of medical experts had serious consequences for the technology and its intended users. As Latour and others have suggested, the fate of technology is in the hands of users (Latour, 1987; Oudshoorn and Pinch, 2003). The boundary work of general practitioners, cardiologists, and heart-failure nurses opened alternative paths for the development of the technology, including a redesign of the telemedical devices. My account of the implementation of the heart mobile phone and the heart-failure telemonitoring system extends Latour's argument further because it shows not only the plasticity of technologies but also the reconfiguration of users. Whereas the heart mobile phone was originally designed for patients, resistance from general practitioners resulted in a situation in which they themselves emerged as primary users. The case of the heart-failure telemonitoring system shows a similar pattern, although resistance was not so much directed to the telecare system as to the telemedical centre that acted as intermediary between healthcare professionals and patients. In contrast to what the innovators expected, the use of a clinical study as implementation strategy did not diminish resistance but reinforced the cardiologists' reluctance to accept the new telecare system. According to the cardiologists, the technology not only disturbed the order of care but also threatened their norms of care. The inter-professional competition between cardiologists, heart-failure nurses, and telecare professionals eventually resulted in a repositioning of the telecare system within the changing landscape of care. Instead of introducing the telemedical centre as an obligatory point of access to the telecare system, the technology was put on the market as a system that also could be used by directly sending patient's data to the heart-failure polyclinic.[9] In this way, cardiologists and heart-failure nurses could keep care of patients in their own hands and the polyclinic would remain the proper place for care provision. Adopting a techno-geographical approach, we can understand these dynamics in terms of a resistance to the new order of care and changes in the spatial dimensions of healthcare inscribed in telecare technologies. The case of the heart-failure–telecare system shows how established medical professionals are not willing to delegate parts of their care work to another category of care workers and another site of care. Instead of passively adopting the redistributions of responsibilities scripted in telecare devices, they forced the new technology to adapt to the existing order of care. Owing to resistance from the medical establishment, promises that telecare technologies would reduce costs in healthcare by delegating tasks to less expensive workers and places will be more difficult to realize.

My analysis of the resistance of healthcare professionals to telecare technologies also shows other dynamics than those described in the literature on boundary work. In contrast to what Abbott and others have described, new technologies not only trigger disputes over the demarcation of boundaries between expert professions but can also lead to contests between professionals and the lay public, in this case patients. The case of the heart mobile phone shows how healthcare professionals resisted the redistribution of responsibilities inscribed by telecare devices by defending their autonomy over the recording of ECGs as against patients who could use the heart mobile phone to make ECGs themselves. The current shift in the political economy of healthcare, in which patients are increasingly being targeted as primary users of all kinds of new medical devices, transforms patients into potential intruders in the domain of general practitioners because the technologies enable them to perform tasks that used to be solely in the hands of the medical profession.

Moreover, the case of the heart mobile phone shows a very specific 'settlement pattern' of boundary work (Gieryn, 1983). The contest between healthcare professionals, on the one hand, and telecare professionals and patients, on the other, was solved not by making specific agreements about how and by whom the technology should be used but by redesigning the new technology. The heart mobile phone was redesigned in such a way that it no longer disturbed the established order of care. By changing the device and its intended user, the new technology became a device that could be incorporated into the domain of the general practitioner and the cardiologist. My analysis thus shows how telecare technologies function as actants that intervene to establish the boundaries of medical professions, in a process in which their own identity is also redefined.

Finally, the case of the heart-failure telemonitoring system shows that boundary work not only involves a defence of professional autonomy – in this case the question of who is qualified to provide medical care to heart-failure patients – but also norms of care. As we have seen, the collaboration among cardiologists, heart-failure nurses, and telecare staff triggered tensions and conflicts about what constitutes good care for heart-failure patients. Chapter 6 investigates the differences in care provided at two competing places of care: the heart-failure polyclinic and the telecare centre. Before turning to these different care practices, the next chapter focuses on telemedical centres and telecare professionals. How do these new places in which healthcare is provided look? Who are these new healthcare workers, and what are their work practices?

Part II
Creating New Forms of Care

5
Telecare Workers: The Invisible Profession

Telecare technologies affect healthcare in a very profound way: they transform its spatial dimensions. Patients no longer have to visit the hospital or the general practitioner's consulting rooms frequently and doctors do not have to pay regular visits to patients' homes to diagnose and monitor chronic diseases because interactions are mediated by ICTs. This does not mean that places no longer matter. Although telecare technologies introduce virtual encounters between healthcare providers and patients, these technology-mediated care practices are always situated somewhere. Drawing on the techno-geographical approach described in Chapter 2, I suggest it is important to take these physical spaces into account in order to understand how telecare technologies transform healthcare. Telecare technologies change the landscape of care not only by distributing care work to familiar places such as hospitals, general practitioners' consulting rooms, and patients' homes, but also by introducing the new spaces of telemedical centres. Most importantly, this spatial reordering of care includes a new category of healthcare providers.

As described in the first chapter, the introduction of telecare technologies produces a proliferation in the care work required to produce, read and interpret more and more diagnostic and monitoring data. This healthcare work is delegated to a variety of actors, including the new category of telecare professionals. Telecare professionals are expected to act as intermediaries among patients, telecare devices, and healthcare professionals. Although popular discourse tries to convince us that telecare technologies require no human work, current telecare technologies depend on specially trained nurses and physicians.

Whereas telecare professionals are expected to play an important role in the changing landscape of healthcare, they are largely invisible.

Telecare workers are rendered invisible in three different ways. First, they are literally invisible because patients and healthcare professionals will never meet them in person. Compared to other healthcare professionals, telecare workers can thus be considered a rather unusual kind of care provider. Whereas traditional healthcare practitioners provide care based on face-to-face contacts with patients, telecare professionals will only deliver healthcare remotely. The novelty and invisibility of their profession makes it rather difficult for telecare professionals to explain to their family and friends what they are actually doing in healthcare.

A second way in which telecare workers are rendered invisible is their absence from formal representations of telecare technologies. As we have seen in Chapter 3, the promises articulated about these new technologies emphasize technological devices rather than the staff of telemedical centres as the agents making care at a distance possible. In contrast to other healthcare professionals, the perspectives and actual work of telecare practitioners are often silenced on websites and other information sources produced by innovators in the field of telemedicine. Spokespersons or pictures of this new category of healthcare worker are absent as well, except for the photos of staff of the telemedical centre in Germany included in the website of the firm. Any discussion of the actual work and care practices of these new healthcare providers is absent from these discourses.

Third, telecare workers, and also telemedical centres, are largely invisible in the literature of medical sociology and science and technology studies (STS). Studies of the consequences of telecare technologies for healthcare work usually focus on traditional healthcare professionals, that is, nurses or doctors in hospitals.[1] This chapter therefore focuses on this new category of healthcare professional and care site. How do these new places in which healthcare is provided remotely look? Who are these new healthcare professionals, and what constitutes their work and care practices? To answer these questions I analyse the care practices of two of the first telemedical centres to deliver healthcare to heart patients in Europe: the telemedical centre run by the Dutch health insurer, Achmea, and the centre operated by the German company Vitaphone, the first and, until now, the only telemedical centre in Germany (Anonymous, 2008). I do not intend to make a systematic comparison between the two centres, but I analyse their different telemedical care practices to provide a more detailed picture of the people and technologies that constitute these novel spaces of care.[2] The first section focuses on gender and the demographic politics involved in staffing the two telemedical centres in Germany and the Netherlands.

In the second and third section, I analyse the role of technologies and boundary work in defining the work practices of telecare workers. In the conclusions I reflect on the kind of healthcare professional that is constituted in telemedical centres.

On women, computers and men

One of the privileges of being a researcher is that you can visit places that are usually not open to the public. When I visited the Vitaphone Medical Service Centre in Chemnitz, Germany, it did not feel like visiting a healthcare organization. The centre looked more like a modern office space dominated by desks with computers. The only clue suggesting a healthcare organization was that the employees watching computer screens were wearing white shirts with the logo *Vitaphone Telemedizin* on the left arm (see Figure 5.1). There was also a man in the room in a white coat, which reflects the professional dress code of healthcare professionals.

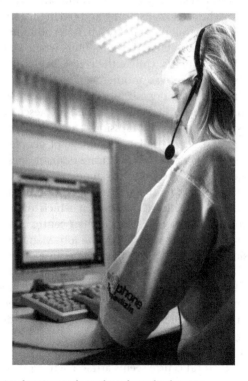

Figure 5.1 White dressing code at the telemedical centre

This confirmed my stereotypical image of healthcare practitioners, but instead of wearing stethoscopes they were wearing headphones. Another striking difference was that patients, or any spaces that indicated visits by patients, such as waiting or consulting rooms, were absent. When I looked around the room, I realized that all the employees working at computers were women (see Figure 3.2).[3] There were only two men standing in a corner, watching the women work. When the director of the medical service centre introduced them to me, I learned that they worked at the centre as physician and supervisor. In this respect there are no differences between this new healthcare organization and traditional organizations. The staffing of the telemedical centre reflects the same gendered hierarchy as other healthcare organizations where men still dominate higher management positions and, to a lesser extent, the profession of physician, whereas women are predominantly employed as nurses or medical assistants.

The Achmea Medical Service Centre in Zwolle, the Netherlands, made a similar impression. Again, a large room dominated by computers and women watching the screens, listening and talking through their headphones, was the scene that presented itself. In a corner hung a big paper sign showing a red heart above the computers where staff was answering calls from heart patients. Unlike the centre in Germany, there were no white coats, but there was another sign that made me aware that I had entered a healthcare organization. On one of the walls I noticed the logo of this telemedical centre that had an Aesculapius in it, the traditional icon of the medical profession. The telemedical centres I visited thus represent a very familiar assemblage of people, symbols, and machines. The newcomer in the healthcare domain does not challenge the existing gendered segregation of labour in the healthcare sector. Instead, this arrangement reinforces the segregation of male and female work by building on gendered patterns in which men dominate the higher segment of professions.[4] The German centre explicitly adopted gender politics by selecting women for the job. Management preferred women, considering them better equipped because of their social competencies, their ability to remain calm and to cope with stress in crisis situations, and because a female voice would be more effective to reassure callers (Interview Murin, 2005). Like nursing, telecare work has thus become a female profession. Historically, the only difference from traditionally gendered patterns of division of labour is perhaps that women's work now includes computer work.[5]

A job at a telemedical centre seems attractive to women who work in the healthcare sector because it offers an alternative to the physically

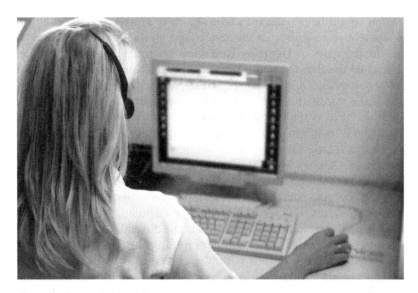

Figure 5.2 A telenurse at work

demanding work involved in providing care at the bedside. Moreover, telemedical centres are based on part-time work, enabling women to combine work and mothering more easily (Interview Sorgdrager, 2006). In the German centre, many women are from single-parent families or provide the major income in the family because their partner is unemployed or has a low income (Interview Murin, 2005).

In addition to gender, there are other demographic politics that shape the composition of the staff of telemedical centres, particularly in Germany. Initially, Vitaphone aimed to establish their first telemedical centre in Mannheim, a city in formerly West Germany, where the firm's director already owned another medical company. This plan could not be realized because it turned out to be very difficult to find physicians willing to work at the telemedical centre. A position at the centre was not attractive to them because they had to work an eight-hour schedule, including night shifts. The telemedical centre operates on the basis of three different shifts to provide continuous service 24 hours a day, 365 days a year (Interview Albani, 2005). Because a centre in Mannheim was thus no longer an option, Vitaphone decided to look for a location in the former East Germany, where they expected it would be easier to interest physicians because of the high unemployment in the eastern regions. Moreover, establishing a centre in this region would be beneficial in terms of costs as well, because the firm could receive a bonus from the national government for hiring employees in this part of Germany (Interview Quinger, and Wittig, 2005). Therefore the first telemedical centre was established in Magdeburg in 2000 (Interview Quinger, 2004). Several years later, a second telemedical centre was established, also in the eastern part of Germany, namely in Chemnitz, in the province of Saxony, in a city formerly known as Karl Marx Stadt.[6] In 2004 the Magdeburg location merged with the Chemnitz location because of the disappointing growth of Vitaphone (Interview Quinger, 2004; Maathuis 2005).

When I visited the telemedical centre in Chemnitz in January 2005, it had a mixed staff composition. The employees answering the calls from patients, referred to as agents ('Agenten' in German), lived in Chemnitz or other villages in the neighbourhood. The director and 60 per cent of the physicians came from the western regions of Germany. The staff of this telemedical centre thus not only reflects a hierarchy according to gender but also in terms of demographic labour politics in which the 'Wessies' (as citizens of former West Germany are called) are positioned higher in the hierarchy of this new organization than the 'Ossies' (citizens of the former East Germany). One of the personnel management policies is to avoid any reinforcement of stereotypical images of the formerly separated German citizens because this 'would ruin the organisation' (Interview Murin, 2005).

Although this historically situated demographic policy involved in staffing is specific for the German centre, both telemedical centres have a hierarchically layered organization of work that includes several functions. First, there are employees responsible for operating the telemonitoring system: the agents (Chemnitz) or medical assistants (the Netherlands). In the remaining text I refer to these employees as telenurses. The second layer consists of a supervisor (Germany) or a team leader (the Netherlands) responsible for the coordination, administration, and organization of training programmes. Third, there are physicians charged with the responsibility of supporting telenurses in difficult cases, to provide medical training (only in Germany), and who have the final responsibility for the quality of the medical services provided by the centres. Finally, the overall responsibility for the centre is delegated to the director and the legal responsibility is charged to the company (Vitaphone in Germany and Achmea in the Netherlands) (Interview Wal, 2006; interview Murin, 2005).

Except for the supervisor and the other managers, most employees have a medical background. Physicians are interns specialized in

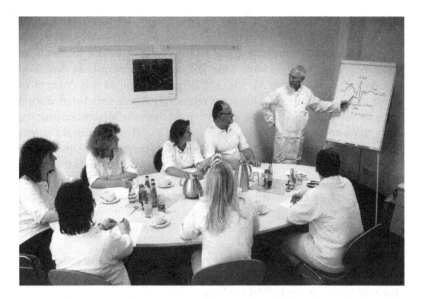

Figure 5.3 Training session at the telemedical centre

cardiology (Germany) or general practitioners (the Netherlands), whereas telenurses are qualified nurses or assistants of general practitioners (the Netherlands), or dieticians (Germany).[7] In addition, telenurses received training to acquire the skills required for operating the software programs used in the centres and attended courses in communication, heart diseases, and (in Germany) reading ECGs and the functioning of Vitaphones' telemonitoring devices (see Figure 5.3).[8]

During the first months of their job, telenurses are also frequently coached by physicians and the supervisor (Interview Murin, 2005; interview Wal, 2006; Achmea Zorg Services, 2006).

The Dutch telemedical centre

Technologies, scripts, and telecare work

Technological objects play a major role in the telemedical centres. The glimpses in the two centres provided above indicate that computer technologies are a key feature of these novel institutional spaces in healthcare. To deliver healthcare remotely, telecare professionals depend on a variety of ICT-based devices. Although computer technologies also assist the work of other healthcare professionals, ICT devices are more consequential for telecare workers because they constitute their entire work practice and profession. Or, even more strongly: telecare technologies are the very reason for the existence of this new healthcare profession. In order to understand how these technologies structure the work of telenurses and telephysicians, I use the concept of script. As described in Chapter 2, Madeleine Akrich (1992) has introduced this concept to make visible how user–technology relations are pre-structured during the process of technological development because designers inscribe their views and expectations concerning the social and political context in which technologies will be used into the contents of the artefact (Akrich, 1992, p. 208). The script approach provides a useful tool for understanding how telecare technologies participate in creating a specific geography of responsibilities between humans and objects by analysing how scripts of technological devices used in telemedical centres delegate actions and responsibilities to telecare workers, patients, and technological devices.

Let us first look at the Dutch telemedical centre. Telecare provided to heart-failure patients by the Achmea medical service centre is based on three different technological devices:

1 a telephone
2 an electronic triage system (TAS) to assess the urgency of health complaints
3 a telemonitoring system, which provides bio-data delivered by patients through electronic devices.

These technological devices enable telecare practitioners to monitor the health condition of heart-failure patients remotely. However, not all the technologies are operated by telenurses or located in the telemedical centre. As described in Chapter 3, the technical devices used to collect bio-data from patients are located in patients' homes. The script of the telemonitoring system is thus not restricted to telecare workers but also includes patients who have to measure their own weight and blood pressure daily by using electronic scales and blood-pressure meters. These measurements are then automatically sent to the telemedical centre. The script of this telecare technology thus delegates the responsibility to initiate the monitoring process to patients and not to healthcare professionals.

Telecare technology concerns three different technological devices. Remarkably, the phone is usually not included in dominant discourses on telecare technologies. Websites, promotion brochures, and policy documents foreground the novel elements of the technology rather than a device that is usually categorized as an 'old media technology'. The contribution of the phone to providing care at a distance is thus taken for granted. Because telecare technology for heart-failure patients consists of multiple technological devices, one cannot talk about 'the' telecare technology because this phrasing hides the complexities of the new technology. In the Dutch telemedical centre, for instance, the successful operation of the heart-failure monitoring technology depends on actions related to three different technical devices. I use the term telecare technology as an overarching term and the term technological devices or systems to refer to each individual technology separately when analysing the scripts of these devices.

To understand how telecare technologies shape the work of telecare professionals it is important to differentiate between the various scripts of the composing technological devices rather than assuming that the telecare technology contains a single, unifying script. I thus adopt a somewhat modified version of the script approach originally developed by Madeleine Akrich (1992) and described in Chapter 2. Most script analyses since Akrich are restricted to a single artefact.[9] Technologies that include multiple artefacts are very interesting for STS because they may involve dynamics of socio-technical change that differ from those of single-artefact technologies. First, technologies that consist of multiple artefacts may imply multiple users, as is exemplified by the telecare technology for heart-failure patients. Patients, telecare workers, and traditional healthcare professionals can all be considered to be users, although their interactions with the telemonitoring technology are not the same, nor are their responsibilities or their positions in the emerging landscape of care. The multiplicity of the telecare technology also triggers new questions about how the technology guides the actions of telecare workers. Not all technological devices may be equally influential in structuring their actions. And, maybe even more importantly, technological devices may also incorporate conflicting guides of action, which complicate the work of their users. In adopting a script approach, we should thus be careful to avoid a phrasing or question, which implies that technologies have a single script. Instead, it seems more useful to differentiate between scripts of the various technological devices that constitute the technology. To understand how the telecare technology guides the actions of telecare workers, I therefore focus on the scripts of the phone, the monitoring system, and the electronic triage system. Are these scripts equally influential in pre-structuring the work of telecare professionals, or are their work practices predominantly defined by the script of one of these technological devices? To what extent do these scripts work together in guiding the work of telecare workers, or are there frictions in these alignments?

In order to understand how and to what extent the scripts of the different technological devices structure and define work practices in the Dutch telemedical centre, I begin my analysis with the first contact between telecare workers and patients. The task to establish this contact is delegated to the monitoring system and not to the phone, which is a major difference from medical call centres, where patients can call healthcare professionals directly. As soon as patients measure their weight and blood pressure, which they are expected to do each day, these measurements are automatically sent to the telemedical centre. Telenurses can watch the results of these measurements on their computer screens. The computer software program of the monitoring system is designed in such a way that it detects differences between the received measurements and the set standards for weight and blood pressure. Patients' biodata should remain within certain limits to prevent a worsening of their health condition. These standards for weight and blood pressure are defined by the treating cardiologist and entered into the telemonitoring system's database by telenurses together with other relevant information about patients, including diagnosis and demographic data, as soon as patients are referred to the telemedical centre (Interview Wal, 2006). Entering data in the telemonitoring database is thus the first task delegated to telenurses. When the monitoring system detects deviating measures, it will give a sign in the shape of a flag, accompanied by the message 'weight too high' or 'blood pressure too high', which appears on the computer screen in the telemedical centre. The responsibility for detecting changes in the health condition of patients is thus delegated to the telemonitoring system.

From this moment onwards, the responsibility for monitoring patients is delegated to telenurses. They are expected to check the box 'Tasks' of the software program daily to see whether and which patients have received a flag signal. When they detect a flag, they have to click the tab-page 'Flag' to check the maximum and minimum values set for the patient's weight and blood pressure. The telemonitoring system provides telecare workers with important information about the health condition of heart-failure patients. To deliver healthcare remotely, they can rely on a systematic and daily overview of patients' weight and blood pressure covering a period of 14 to 30 days, which is shown in the form of a graph on their computer screens (Achmea Zorg Services, 2006). The monitoring system also provides telenurses with a regime for nurse–patient interactions. The script of the system urges nurses to watch their computer screens regularly to notice warnings of deviating measures and to call patients as soon as a warning is detected. Telenurses thus have to switch to using the phone. They are expected to phone the patient to enquire about the cause of their increased weight or blood pressure (Interview Borst and Sorgdrager, 2006). The phone call to patients is structured along three leading questions: 'How are you doing at the moment?' 'Has anything changed in the past few days?' 'Are there any changes in your medication?' (Achmea Zorg Services 2006, p. 17). Telenurses are also expected to call the heart-failure polyclinic to change the medication required to stabilize blood pressure or reduce weight. The script of the telemonitoring system thus relies heavily on the use of the telephone.

In order to align the use of the phone to the script of the monitoring system, telenurses have to insert a reminder in the telemonitoring software program that they should not forget to call patients with deviating measures. Phone calls to patients are not restricted to a one-time occasion but usually involve more frequent contacts in which telenurses enquire how patients are doing (Interview Borst and Sorgdrager 2006). As soon as patients use the telecare technology, they can call the telemedical centre by themselves as well. The interactions between telenurse and patients are thus not one-directional. The telemedical centre therefore distinguishes between two kinds of phone contacts with patients: 'outbound calls' in the case where a telenurse calls patients, and 'inbound calls', when patients initiate phone calls themselves (Achmea Zorg Services, 2006, p. 10). Patients who use the telemonitoring system can call the telemedical centre with a request for medical assistance or questions concerning their diet or medication, or health complaints that may not necessarily be related to heart failure, which might require referral to the treating physician or, when a matter is urgent, the hospital.

Compared to the telemonitoring system, the phone has a rather weak script in terms of guiding the actions of nurses. When used as a separate device, the phone does not put any constraints on the actions of its users, except that it is restricted to supporting verbal communication – at least that is the case with the phone used in this telemedical centre. The responsibility for structuring the calls is delegated to another technological device: the triage advice system TAS[10] (Achmea Zorg Services, 2006, p. 11). Similarly to other electronic triage systems used in medical call centres and hospitals elsewhere in Europe, Canada and the US, TAS provides a strict protocol that nurses have to follow to ensure a uniform approach to processing a call. The TAS system is designed to determine the urgency of a complaint and answer requests for medical assistance. It consists of protocols to guide interventions and provides information about symptoms of diseases (Achmea Zorg Services, 2006, p. 14). The use of TAS in the Dutch telemedical centre can be considered as an additional technological device. The original design of the telemonitoring technology for heart-failure patients did not include a separate triage system but relied only on the monitoring of biodata and phone-mediated contacts between patients, telenurses, and traditional healthcare professionals. Nevertheless, Achmea decided to include the triage advice system in operating the telemonitoring system, partly because the employees of their medical service centre were already used to working with this system when answering calls from users of the other health services provided by the centre. Consequently, telenurses could be more easily appointed to the new task of answering the calls of heart-failure patients. A more important reason, however, was that the use of TAS provided the healthcare insurer with a tool with which to legitimate the decisions and advice of telecare workers where cases of juridical claims related to accusations of inadequate care arose (Interview Wal, 2006). Obviously, Achmea put more trust in a system they were already familiar with than in the new telemonitoring system.

When a patient calls for medical assistance, the telenurse on duty has to check the patient's demographic information included in the database of the telemonitoring system and check the information about the patient's medical history under the tab-page 'Overview'. The telenurse is then expected to shift to the TAS software program to assess the patient's health problem and the urgency of the complaint. The electronic triage system is not a diagnostic tool. The system is designed to collect information from patients in order to assess the urgency (or acuity) of the complaint. The script of the system is that it generates the relevant questions that telenurses should ask patients to determine or clarify their complaints. The script thus delegates agency to telenurses (they should ask questions and enter data in the system), but the control over which questions are relevant to address is delegated to the software program. The system is designed in such a way that it maps patients' complaints to specific locations in the body, specific items and questions, and urgency scores. For example, when patients call the medical service centre with a complaint about pressure on their chest, the telenurse has to select the organ related to the complaint from a list shown on the tab-page Anamnesis, in this case 'chest'. The triage system then automatically provides a list of items and questions telenurses should address in the further conversation with the patient. Telenurses have to enter the answer to these questions in the fields connected to the items and have to fill in all the fields before they can continue with the next page of the anamnesis (Spelten and Gubbels, 2003, p. 545). Sometimes the triage system will display a pop-up with an additional question telenurses should ask patients to assess a complaint.

When telenurses have completed all the items, the electronic triage system generates an acuity score that is shown in numbers and colours varying from ten and dark red to one and light green. A high number and dark red indicates that the patients' complaint should be considered urgent and requires immediate, possibly emergency care. Based on the urgency score, telenurses have to contact the heart-failure polyclinic, advise patients to contact their general practitioner, or give advice concerning diet or lifestyle (Achmea Zorg Services, 2006). In case of doubt, they can consult the telephysician who supervises their work, which they do by raising a red or green card above their head to attract the physician's attention (Interview Balk, 2005). The electronic triage system thus incorporates a very forceful script that largely delegates responsibility for assessing patients' complaints to the technological device. By applying standardized categories for action, the system determines how telenurses should act according to rules and protocols built into the system.[11]

Abstract rationality, managerial politics, and boundary work

Together with the telemonitoring system, the electronic triage system thus imposes a structure that defines how telenurses are supposed to work. The scripts of these technological devices constitute telecare work as highly pre-structured and protocol-driven. Although the emergence of these scripts is not the focus of my analysis, we may wonder why the actions scripted in the technological devices leave almost no room for the responsibility, expertise, and tacit knowledge of nurses. Although engineers play an important role in developing technologies and scripts may thus be related to their technological choices, scripts can also emerge because of the policies of other actors. As MacKay et al. (2000) have described, engineers are often constrained by the management of their organization. The TAS triage system is a case in point, although the script of the system does not originate from the engineering organizations McKay described but is related to the politics of healthcare organizations. Electronic triage systems such as TAS reflect a managerial perspective on providing healthcare in which management aims to objectify and treat as routine the procedures for healthcare work. Because of the shift towards the neo-liberalization and modernization of healthcare described in the first chapter, healthcare management has come to rely increasingly on protocols and standards to ensure discipline and control over the work of healthcare professionals. One of the ways in which management can achieve control over labour is through technology. Electronic triage systems are one example of a variety of technological subsystems, often ICT-based, that have been introduced recently to standardize and objectify medical work.[12]

One consequence of this shift towards neo-liberalization and modernization of healthcare is that medical work has become increasingly based on a reductionist view of health. As the electronic triage system shows, the technological device forces telenurses to seek single answers to the often complex health complaints of heart-failure patients.[13] This approach to healthcare relies on an abstract rationality in which following standardized protocols has become the dominant way to determine what is wrong with patients (Berg, 1997; Hanlon, 2005; Townly, 2002).

In my analysis I use the notion of abstract rationality as described by Townly, who used the term to refer to a form of knowledge that objectivizes and treats as routine procedures of labour (Townley, 2002). Similarly to what Giddens has observed for other expert systems, telemonitoring and electronic triage systems incorporate and reinforce ways of knowing that are disembedded and abstracted from a context (Giddens, 1991). The script of the TAS electronic triage system reflects a similar reliance on abstract rationality: it imposes on work a structure that leaves no room for expertise or the tacit knowledge of telecare workers. The design of this technological device thus shows how managers invest more trust in the abstract rationality of a system than in the expertise of professionals (in this case nurses).[14]

The scripts of the telecare technology for heart-failure patients are, however, shaped not only by the managerial political agenda of the neo-liberalization and modernization of healthcare. Some technological choices, particularly about the monitoring system, are clearly related to the boundary work of traditional healthcare professionals. As described in the previous chapter, the implementation of the heart-failure telecare technology faced resistance from cardiologists who refused to delegate part of their responsibility to telecare professionals. This boundary work resulted in a situation in which telecare workers were not allowed to change medication. Consequently, the telemonitoring system was designed in such a way that telenurses should contact heart-failure nurses at polyclinic to request changes in medication. This script thus reduces the responsibility that could be delegated to telecare professionals. The geography of responsibility between heart-failure polyclinics and the telemedical centre shows a strict distribution of tasks in which the responsibility for monitoring the health condition and giving advice about diet and lifestyle are delegated to the telecare nurses, whereas responsibility for medical interventions, including medication, remains restricted to heart-failure nurses and cardiologists (Interview Wal, interview heart-failure nurse A, 2007).

The main responsibility for healthcare thus remains firmly entrenched in the hands of traditional healthcare professionals. As one of the heart-failure nurses described this hierarchy in the emerging landscape of telecare:

> You should not compare telenurses with heart-failure nurses. They are nurses behind a phone and a computer who select for me what is important.
>
> (Interview heart-failure nurse A, 2006)

Telenurses are thus expected to provide services to support the work of cardiologists and heart-failure nurses (Achmea Zorg Services, 2006, p. 3). The protocol of collaboration between the medical service centre and the heart-failure polyclinic also reflects this hierarchical relationship between telenurses and traditional healthcare professionals. It includes an agreement that the heart-failure polyclinic will evaluate the adequacy of the actions of telenurses within 24 hours after each interaction between telenurses and patients (Achmea Zorg Services, 2006, p. 5).

Practical rationality and work-arounds

As we have seen, technologies play an important role in defining the work of telecare professionals. But although technologies may be designed to structure telemedical work, they can never completely control human action. Following Akrich and Latour, who argued that users may resist or modify scripts, it seems likely that telecare workers will not passively follow the actions or accept the responsibilities inscribed in telecare technologies: users may develop anti-programmes. Technologies that contain multiple artefacts and scripts may grant even more flexibility to users: they can resist the script of one of the technological devices because they can rely on one of the other scripts. In this respect, Gasser's notion of 'work-around' provides a useful concept to understand how and whether users will accept certain scripts but reject others. Gasser introduced this concept to refer to situations in which people 'avoid a computer's use ... and rely on an alternative means of accomplishing work' (Gasser, 1986, p. 216). As Bowker and

Star (1999) have argued, technologies that rely on abstract rationality can never entirely capture what is important in providing care. Technological devices that aim to reduce the subjectivity of labour may trigger work-arounds on the part of their users. Healthcare professionals may thus resist the pre-structured and protocol-driven work inscribed in technological systems because they prefer to rely on their own expertise and tacit knowledge and want to take responsibility for providing care by themselves. Instead of passively adopting the abstract, standardized knowledge of the technological devices, they may choose to rely on what Hanlon has called 'practical rationality'. Practical rationality refers to 'knowledge that is context specific, local, located in a social setting and built around a specific, not generalized, other' (Hanlon et al., 2005, p. 150). A reliance on practical rationality implies that telenurses may value their experience and context-specific, often tacit knowledge over the abstract knowledge embedded in the technological devices they have to use to deliver healthcare remotely.

Work practices at the Dutch telemedical centre indicate that managers are very well aware of the limitations of the protocol-driven, standardized technological devices used in the centre. The team leader of this centre emphasized that it is crucial that telecare workers have a medical background because these technologies cannot be operated by employees who are only experienced in working with computers. Although the technological devices provide highly pre-structured and protocol-driven procedures of work, the employees who operate the system have to rely on their medical expertise because they have to know how to interpret the pre-structured questions provided by the system as well as the answers of patients. The telemedical centre's personnel policy is therefore aimed explicitly at hiring qualified nurses to operate the technologies (Interview Wal, 2006). The telephysician responsible for supervising and supporting telenurses was initially rather sceptical about using the electronic triage system:

> I was very sceptical because I had seen similar programs. Therefore I was sceptical but that has changed because the training made us more familiar with the system. But all of us who began to work with this system initially wondered whether and how this would work. How should we make a decision about the urgency of a complaint only based on this system?
>
> (Interview Borst, 2006)

Although this scepticism seems to have largely disappeared after the special skills training employees at the centre received before they started their jobs, practices at the telemedical centre indicate that telecare workers developed work-arounds while using the system. Instead of flying blind on the scripts of the technological devices, telenurses often trusted their own practical rationality over the abstract knowledge of the systems. As Hanlon observed of telenurses at the NHS-Direct medical call centre in the UK, telecare professionals continue to value their own expertise and tacit knowledge, although they use their practical rationality selectively (Hanlon, 2005, p. 158, 159).[15]

The use of both the electronic triage system and the telemonitoring system show instances in which telenurses prioritized their own practical knowledge. While using the telemonitoring system, telenurses often ignore frequent flags, which signal that patients have exceeded the set standards of weight and blood pressure. When they receive frequent flags, usually about weight, they do not follow the script of the system that tells them to call the patient to find out what is wrong. They may do this once or twice but when the system continues to send warnings they will call the heart-failure polyclinic to ask the nurse to change patient's limits for weight. They do this because they expect that the patient will not change his or her behaviour and the system will therefore continue to send warnings every day. As described in the previous chapter, heart-failure nurses do not always agree to change the standards, but sometimes they do. Telenurses can resist the frequent flags because they can switch to the phone. By using the phone, telenurses can become familiar with the specific contexts of patients, that is, their willingness and ability to adhere to the strict regime of lifestyle and medication. Telenurses value this practical knowledge medicated by the phone over the abstract knowledge inscribed in the telemonitoring system that does not differentiate among patients' attitudes towards disciplining their behaviour. In the abstract rationality of the monitoring system, a flag is a flag and can disappear only when the condition of the patient has returned within the set limits of weight because of changed medication or behaviour. In the practical rationality of telenurses, flags may require different actions for different patients. For some patients it may imply changing medication, for others it may require a further fine-tuning of the set standard for weight. Telenurses thus try to overcome one of the constraints of the script of the telemonitoring system by relying on their own practical knowledge. Most importantly, they could develop a work-around because the telephone provided an alternative to the script of the telemonitoring system.

As with the telemonitoring system, telenurses also developed a work-around in relation to the script of the electronic triage system. Work practices at the Dutch telemedical centre show how telecare workers often do not accept the system's evaluation of the urgency of the complaints of the caller. As one of the nurses explained her use of the system:

> When you receive a call from someone who feels tight in the chest you open the box of breathing problems [the nurse points to the computer screen. N. O.]. Then a series of questions will be shown and you will pose these questions and then it will give you a score. That score is not always ... uh ... this program has not been developed to monitor heart-failure but for emergency cases. When it becomes red, it is urgent, but that is not necessarily the case for heart-failure patients ... although, yes, when it becomes really bright red, it will be red, but sometimes it shows red or not-red when it should have done that.
>
> (Interview Sorgdrager, 2006)

The physician at the telemedical centre voiced a similar criticism of the computer system. Because TAS is designed to assess acute situations and chronic heart failure is a chronic disease, the system usually gives too strong an evaluation of the urgency of the call. Here we see how the script of one technological device is not aligned with the script of another device. Whereas TAS may tell nurses that the patient's condition requires immediate medical assistance, the telemonitoring system assesses the situation as less urgent because it concerns a chronic patient. Therefore telecare workers use the electronic triage system not as a tool to assess the urgency of calls but as a checklist (Interview Borst and Sorgdrager, 2006).

Although TAS may not seem to be an appropriate software program to assess the calls of heart-failure patients, the telemedical centre has chosen to use the system, not only because of the legal and skills reasons described above, but also because they consider it as a tool for reducing uncertainty and countering a lack of self-confidence. As the telephysician put it:

> We use TAS because ... In the beginning, we all had the feeling that we were just becoming involved with heart-failure, independently of whether you could rely on previous experience or not. Often it is already several years ago, so we use TAS for our own feeling of safety: to make sure that you do not miss anything, and also

as a checklist. There are always specific questions you have to ask heart-failure patients. By now we do not actually need this anymore because these questions are all here [the physician points at her head. N.O.] because you have posed them so often. But even then it is good to check [them]. Also, in case of doubt, because in difficult cases you can check whether TAS gives the red signal. In that case you take a certainty for an uncertainty.

(Interview Borst, 2006)

Although TAS thus assists nurses to cope with uncertainty, nurses still rely on their own experience. To quote one of the nurses again:

The system does not provide a diagnosis. It only gives me an indication of urgency. Based on this indication I will consult others; it will remain your own assessment.

(Interview Sorgdrager, 2006)

These practices at the Dutch telemedical centre thus exemplify how telenurses often continue to value or sometimes even prioritize their own experience and their colleagues' expertise over the abstract, codified knowledge of the electronic triage system. Equally importantly, these practices show how telecare professionals could develop work-arounds to ignore this part of the script of the electronic triage system because they could rely on the phone to accomplish their work. Or as the telephysician explained how she gained self-confidence in answering the calls of heart-failure patients:

My confidence is based on experience and education. I do not trust the TAS system in itself. I can answer a call without using the system, but I need it to do the paper work. What patients tell you on the phone is very important; that counts for 80 to 90 per cent. And of course it is very convenient to have objective data on weight and blood pressure provided by the telemonitoring system in addition. But without it I can find my way as well. It is a nice, additional tool, particularly to communicate with the cardiologist in the hospital and the patient, so it is a communication device. But without the telemonitoring system we can do the job as well, to put it bluntly.

(Interview Borst, 2006)

In the context of the Dutch telemedical centre, the electronic triage system and the telemonitoring system thus become transformed into communication technologies rather than technologies that assist with the assessment of the health condition of patients. Nurses trust more what they can hear by phone than what they can see on the computer screen. Their ways of knowing thus value the patient's account of symptoms over a systematic assessment of complaints guided by digital technological devices. As is described in the next chapter, there are more instances in which telenurses prioritize their own practical knowledge over the abstract rationality of the technological systems.

The German telemedical centre

Technologies, scripts, and telecare work

Like heart-failure telemonitoring technology, the heart mobile phone, one of the telecare services provided by the Vitaphone Medical Service Centre in Chemnitz, Germany, consists of multiple artefacts. To deliver healthcare remotely, the employees at this telemedical centre have to operate two different technological devices:

1 a telephone
2 a telemonitoring data system, which includes ECGs delivered by patients through the heart mobile phone.

Both technological devices play an important role in defining and structuring the work of telecare staff, particularly the work of telenurses. As we have seen in the Dutch telemedical centre, the task of operating the telecare technology in the telemedical centre is largely delegated to telenurses. Although telephysicians and supervisors are also charged with the responsibility for deliver care remotely, basic actions are performed by telenurses. To paraphrase the situation in regular hospitals where tasks related to working 'at the bedside' are delegated to nurses, the division of labour in telemedical centres can best be captured by the metaphor 'at the computer side'. Although there are similarities between working at the bedside and the computer side, namely that both images refer to proximity to patients, there is a major difference as well. Nurses' work at the bedsides of patients in hospitals is an integral part of a care trajectory in which other healthcare professionals usually take the lead, but telenurses' work at the computer side enables them to initiate the care trajectory. The computer-side metaphor is also useful in describing the spatial dimension of the division of labour that characterizes telemedical centres, where telenurses' work is bound to a computer desk, where they are expected to perform basic tasks to deliver care remotely. In contrast, the work of telephysicians and supervisors is not confined to one specific location. They are expected to support and supervise telenurses by moving around in the office space or performing administrative duties in a separate room. Despite the centrality of telenurses' actions, their work is usually silenced in the dominant discourses on telecare technologies. As described in Chapter 3, Vitaphone is doing a better job than the two other telemedical firms analysed in this book: telecare workers are well represented on the German firm's website, including pictures of the staff of the telemedical centre in Chemnitz, thus giving a face to these invisible professionals. One of these pictures, where a male telephysician bends over the shoulder of a female telenurse to watch her computer screen, captures visually the spatial, and also gendered, division of labour in a nutshell. Telenurses work at the computer side whereas telephysicians, who can move freely around in the office, supervise their work (see Figure 5.4).

Let us take a closer look at how the technical devices available to telenurses shape their work. What actions are inscribed in the devices, and how do their scripts collaborate or compete in defining and structuring the work of telenurses? As with the heart-failure telemonitoring system, the task of establishing the first contact between telenurses and patients is delegated to the patients. When patients experience heart

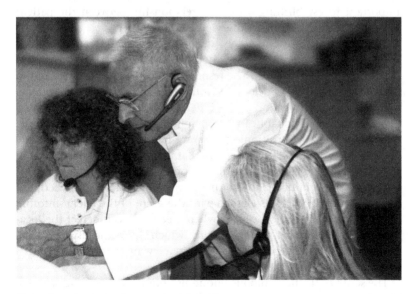

Figure 5.4   A telephysician supervising telenurses

problems, they can register an ECG and send it to the telemedical centre by pressing a button on their heart mobile phone. Patients can also contact the medical service centre by pressing the emergency button to ask for assistance with receiving immediate medical care (Interview Sack, 2004). When a patient contacts the telemedical centre, the telenurse on duty will see a pop-up on her computer screen that informs her about the call and the kinds of telemonitoring device used by the caller. Because callers can use mobile phones with different functionalities (a cardiophone, an emergency phone, and a three-button phone), identifying the type of mobile phone is important for the telenurses who answer and process the calls (Maathuis, 2005). The software of the telemonitoring system is designed in such a way that it identifies the caller automatically because of a special identification number based on the mobile phone number of the patient. When a patient calls the telemedical centre, the database of the telemonitoring system will be opened immediately. The database includes demographic data and relevant medical data entered by telenurses as soon as a patient has purchased a cardiophone. The responsibility of identifying the caller and to select patients' data is thus delegated to the telemonitoring system and not to the telenurse. This technological choice simplifies telenurses' work because they immediately know who is calling. This script enables telenurses to welcome the caller personally by name, which is considered important to establishing a trusting relationship between the patient and the telemedical centre (Interview Sack, 2004).

To deliver healthcare remotely, telenurses cannot rely only on automatic identification of the caller; they also have to rely on an identification of the caller's location. The responsibility to identify callers and to locate their position is delegated to the patient's heart mobile phone. Whereas the identification of the caller is enabled by a special number given to each individual heart mobile phone number, the caller can be located by the GPS positioning software built in to the cardiophone. The phone is designed in such a way that it automatically transmits the GPS data to the telemedical centre as soon as a patient contacts the centre by pressing a button on his or her heart mobile phone. This script of the heart mobile phone is aligned with the script of the telemonitoring system at the telemedical centre, where telenurses can detect the location of the caller on a map of Germany, which shows the city or village, the neighbourhood, and the street within a few metres from the caller's position (Vitaphone, 2006).

The script of the heart mobile phone also prescribes two other actions: the recording and transmission of ECGs. Both actions are delegated to the phone, although the responsibility for initiating the recording of ECGs is delegated to patients. Again, the heart mobile phone and the telemonitoring data system are designed in such a way that their scripts collaborate smoothly to support the provision of healthcare at a distance. When patients send an ECG by their heart mobile phone, a graphic representation of the ECG is automatically shown on the telenurse's computer screen (Murin, 2005). Although most attention is usually given to the ECG-transmitting action of the cardiophone, an equally important part of the script is that it enables communication between the caller and telecare professionals. This communication is structured by the script of the telemonitoring system. As mentioned above, the telemonitoring system informs telenurses about a caller by a pop-up on their computer screen. The opening page of the database automatically shows the personal data of the patient, with tabs indicating the contents of the other pages, as well as a short note on the specific situation of the caller. The database stores patients' personal data, an overview of previous calls, the disease history, ECGs, anamnesis, information on medication and allergies, information about the mobile phone, the addresses and phone numbers of next of kin, the contact data of the treating physician, and an overview of all relevant data to be used in case of emergencies (Murin, 2005, p. 9). Telenurses are responsible for entering or changing these data based on information provided by patients during a phone call, although some information, such as ECGs and an overview of previous calls, is stored automatically. The script of the telemonitoring system thus delegates the responsibility for collecting and selecting relevant information from phone conversations with patients and documenting this information in the database to telenurses. They are also expected to read the received ECGs, although the final responsibility for evaluating ECGs is delegated to telephysicians. Moreover, telenurses have to forward relevant information from a patient's call to the treating doctor and, in the case of an emergency, call an ambulance and forward information to the hospital to which the patient is admitted (Vitaphone, 2006, p. 9). Finally, telenurses are also responsible for giving instructions to patients when they face problems in using the mobile phone and for testing Vitaphone's health mobile phones, that is, checking batteries and the overall functioning of the phones (Interview Gahlert, 2005).

The work of telenurses in the German telemedical centre is thus rather similar to the work of their Dutch colleagues, except for assessing ECGs and testing mobile phones. In both centres, telenurses' work is largely defined and structured by the use of digital technological systems, which contain rather strict scripts. As in the Dutch telemedical centre, German telenurses have to fill in all the fields of the telemonitoring data system before the system allows them to continue to the next page. If they do not follow this part of the script, the system will give them an alarm notice to tell them they should add the missing data (Interview Gahlert, 2005). Telenurses' work can thus be considered as highly pre-structured and protocol-driven work based on the abstract rationality inscribed in these technological systems. However, there are major differences between the German and the Dutch telemedical centres. Whereas telenurses' work in the Netherlands, in addition to the phone, depends on two digital technological devices (a telemonitoring system and an electronic triage system), the work of telenurses in Germany is structured only by a telemonitoring system. The German telemedical centre thus delegates more responsibility to telenurses because there is no strict protocol for processing phone calls. German telenurses can rely on an electronic handbook, a kind of helpdesk, that includes information about procedures to process calls, medical information, and instruction guides for the mobile phones, but this handbook does not control their actions (Interview Murin, 2005).

Work practices at the German telemedical centre also allow more flexibility in telephysicians' work. The script for the phone enables telephysicians to act more independently of the telemonitoring system. The phone includes a conference system that supports a phone conversation by three parties: the patient, the telenurse, and the telephysician. During their training telenurses learn that they should always seek the assistance of a telephysician in case of doubt or in difficult cases. In such a situation, the telenurse has to inform the patient that the telephysician on duty will join the phone conversation and has to switch on the three-party conference system. The telenurse will notify the physician by standing up, which alerts the physician to the telenurse who is seeking assistance. The physician then joins the conversation by using his headphone and the nurse briefly informs him about the patient's complaint. The telephysician will then open the telemonitoring data system on his desk where he can view the patient's disease history, or review previous calls or other relevant data. Then he will take over the phone conversation with the patient from the nurse. The telenurse is expected to document the contents of the conversation in the database (Interview Murin, 2005). The way in which difficult cases are processed exemplifies the division of labour between telenurses and telephysicians already described above. Most importantly, it shows how the script of the phone enables telephysicians to work around the pre-structured actions of the telemonitoring system, a flexibility that is not granted to telenurses. The use of the phone thus facilitates a situation in which the telephysician can ask questions to assess patients' complaints; and he can rely on his own practical knowledge based on previous experience with similar cases (Interview Wittig, 2005). Telenurses are also expected to seek the physician's assistance if they notice irregularities in the ECGs forwarded by patients. Although telenurses have learned to 'read' ECGs and have acquired the skills to detect heart-rhythm disturbances, some rhythm irregularities are difficult to detect and require the expertise of the physician (Interview Albani, 2005).[16] When this happens, the physician will ask the patient to send another ECG and he will make his own assessment (Interview Gahlert, 2005).

The work practices at the German telemedical centre indicate that telecare work is thus not necessarily individual work, as is sometimes suggested in studies of how ICT systems structure the work of healthcare professionals.[17] Although work at the German telemedical centre consists for the most part of individual work, particularly by telenurses, there are also instances of teamwork where telenurses, supervisors, and telephysicians collaborate to deliver care remotely. Because telenurses and supervisors can always rely on the assistance of telephysicians, they feel more reassured to handle difficult calls. To quote one of the supervisors:

> In the beginning we thought what should we do in case of an emergency? We were all very much afraid ['himmelangst' in German; N. O.]. But when it happened, we experienced how everything works together. I lost my fears when I saw how the call circulated over the different places and how everybody collaborated to deal with it ... Now it has become a routine. We all got used to each other's ways.
>
> (Interview Albani, 2005)

When telenurses receive difficult calls or become nervous because of aggressive calls, they can rely on the supervisor, who will come to their desk to calm them, which is usually done by putting a hand on the shoulder. Telenurses may also experience sexual intimidation by callers; when this happens, they are allowed to end the phone conversation (Interview Albani, 2005). Eye contact or making faces to other telenurses, or standing up to draw the attention of the supervisor, are also used to release stress when telenurses become irritated by aggressive or intimidating calls. The supervisor can overhear the phone calls at his own desk when nurses request his assistance. Mutual support and collaboration thus plays an important role in telecare work, particularly in reducing the stress of telenurses' work.

Bypassing and rejecting scripts

Although work at the German telemedical centre can thus be characterized as highly pre-structured and protocol-driven, this does not imply that telecare workers passively follow the scripts of the technical devices used in this centre. As at the Dutch telemedical centre, work practices at the German telemedical centre show how telecare workers develop work-arounds in which they bypass the script of one technological device by relying on another device. Although transmitting ECGs by mobile phone is the major novelty of the cardiophone, and it thus seems likely that this part of the script will structure the actions of telecare workers, they do not always follow this script. As the director of the telemedical centre explained:

> In addition to the ECG we have verbal communication with the customer. When there is a customer who tells us that he has so much pressure on his chest that it feels as if there is an elephant sitting on it, we do not ask him to send an ECG, even if he uses a cardiophone. Then we seek the assistance of the telephysician immediately and he tries to describe the symptoms in as much detail as possible. We do not depend on an ECG then.
>
> (Interview Murin, 2005)

The telephysician explained this bypassing of the ECG in similar terms. According to the telephysician, the ECG is a matter of secondary importance, at least in those cases in which patients have previously been diagnosed with a heart attack. Practices at the telemedical centre thus show how telecare staff could work around the ECG part of the script of the telemonitoring system by relying on the phone: they sometimes prioritize information from verbal communication with patients provided by phone contacts over information provided by ECGs. The communication script of the phone enables telecare workers to have access to the contextual, situated knowledge of patients, which provides important information to assess patients' heart problems. ECGs are thus constituted as an optional rather than an obligatory passage point to deliver healthcare remotely, at least to patients with previous heart attacks, who are considered as a major audience for the heart mobile phone. But even in cases of heart-attack survivors, telecare workers do not ignore the ECG. Telenurses in training at the German telemedical centre are instructed not to jump to conclusions too quickly when an ECG shows no irregularities. Patients who previously experienced a heart attack may show a 'normal' ECG, particularly in the acute phase (Interview Wittig, 2005).

Work practices at the German telemedical centre not only reveal how telecare workers bypass the script of the telemonitoring system; they also show how they reject the restricted agency delegated to telephysicians in the assessment of heart complaints. These restrictions are not inscribed in the technology but in legal regulations.

As we have seen in the previous chapter, telecare professionals are not allowed to make diagnoses because this task is restricted to traditional healthcare practitioners. According to German law, healthcare professionals who do not know the patient personally are not entitled to treat or diagnose patients by phone (Interview Murin, 2005). The task of telecare workers is to make an assessment of the patient's complaint and forward this information to the treating doctor. Nevertheless, telephysicians often make a diagnosis or, to quote the telephysician again:

> We do not make a diagnosis but an assessment. We have discussed this many times, because we are not allowed to make a diagnosis. Being a physician I always make a summary, I have to characterize an emergency situation and of course I have my own thoughts about the underlying cause of the complaint. I have a diagnosis in the back of my mind. I cannot do it in another way. I have to have a working hypothesis. Therefore I always resist when they say that we are not allowed to make diagnoses.
>
> (Interview Wittig, 2005)

The telephysician thus tries to challenge established divisions of tasks and responsibilities with traditional healthcare professionals. The German centre legitimates this resistance by arguing that it is in the interests of the patient to receive immediate care in cases of emergency. A preliminary diagnosis may facilitate and accelerate adequate care. Equally importantly, healthcare professionals contacted by the telemedical centre also expect to be informed about the possible cause of their complaint (Interview Wittig, 2005). This practice at the telemedical centre thus indicates how telecare workers and traditional healthcare professionals bypass the formal division of tasks.

Telecare professionals thus perform various work-arounds to deliver healthcare remotely. However, they are not alone in resisting the scripts of the technology. As telecare workers, patients also try to modify or resist the actions delegated to them by the telecare technology. Although patients' actions are discussed more extensively in the last two empirical chapters of this book, I describe one specific kind of activity here because this is relevant to understanding how technologies shape the work of healthcare professionals. As described above, patients are expected to call the telemedical centre only to send ECGs or to ask questions about the outcome of the ECG or problems related to their heart complaint. However, some patients do not adhere to this script. Telenurses sometimes receive phone calls from people who are psychologically derailed or suffer from dementia. Other people may call the centre but keep silent. These kinds of call may occur once a day on average. In such situations, telenurses will usually contact family members of the caller to inform them what happened. This may mean that a patient's relative will take away a parent's mobile phone to prevent further 'misuse' (Interview Albani, 2005). At the German telemedical centre, the staff is instructed to end these kinds of phone call within three seconds when they receive more urgent calls. Nevertheless, they are also expected to remain calm and friendly and learn to consider these calls as part of their job (Interview Albani, 2005; Interview Murin, 2005). As described for medical call centres in the UK, callers thus may seek interactions that are not scripted in the telecare technology, simply because they want to talk to someone (Hanlon et al., 2005). Work practices in the German centre indicate how balancing patients' needs for contact against constraints on interactions inscribed in the telecare technology is an important part of telecare work.

Conclusions: The intermediary profession

Reflecting on my analysis of work practices at the Dutch and German telemedical centre, what can we conclude about the kind of healthcare professional created in these novel organizations? To answer this question I first summarize what structures their work. Perhaps not very surprisingly, technologies turn out to be major actors in defining and structuring telecare work. My analysis shows how telecare work largely depends on and is defined by various technological devices. The scripts of telemonitoring devices, the phone, and (in the Netherlands) an electronic triage system constitute telecare work as highly pre-structured and protocol-driven. Although technologies are increasingly important in shaping healthcare work in general, technological devices constitute the entire work practice of telecare workers. The healthcare professional created in telemedical centres is disciplined to prioritize the objective, standardized knowledge scripted in technological devices over personal and practical knowledge. However, there is also an important similarity with other healthcare work: both telecare and traditional healthcare show an increased reliance on procedures that are objective and rendered routine, which reflects the shift towards neo-liberalization and modernization in healthcare that aims to standardize and control healthcare work in general.

Although ICT-based technologies impose a structure upon the working telecare providers, the technical devices included in telecare technologies are not equally influential in pre-structuring and defining this work. By modifying the script approach, in which I argued that it is important to acknowledge that technologies may consist of multiple artefacts and contain multiple scripts, I could show how some technological devices have scripts that are more forceful than others. Of the technological devices that constitute telecare technologies, the telemonitoring system (in Germany and the Netherlands) and the electronic triage system (in the Netherlands) have the most compelling scripts. Both systems impose actions upon telenurses in such a way that they cannot escape the script for collecting and entering data. If telenurses do not fill in all the fields of the electronic data systems, the system does not allow them to continue to the next page of the protocol. Compared to the telemonitoring systems and the electronic triage system, the phone reveals a less rigid script. Although it is meant to be used in a certain way, actors can more easily escape the script because the prescribed actions are not inscribed in this technological device but in additional guidelines. Both telemedical centres have instructions for telenurses (an electronic handbook in Germany and paper protocols in the Netherlands) that tell them how they should handle or process calls. There is, however, no feedback system or barrier built in to the phone that corrects them if they do not follow these instructions. The structuring of phone calls is not delegated to the phone but to the telemonitoring system, and, in the Netherlands, to the electronic triage system. In this respect, there are important differences between the so-called old and new communication technologies. The phone, as a representative of the generation of communication technologies prior to the introduction of ICT-based communication technologies, grants more responsibility and control to telecare workers than the new communication technologies, that is, the telemonitoring and the electronic triage system.

My focus on the multiplicity of artefacts and scripts also enabled me to investigate the extent to which scripts of technological devices work together to structure telecare work, or whether there are frictions in these alignments. Technologies consisting of multiple artefacts may give more flexibility to users: they can bypass the script of one particular device because they can rely on the scripts of the other devices. This may be even easier when there is no alignment between the devices. My analysis shows several instances of work-arounds, where telecare workers could bypass part of the script of one of the technical devices because they could rely on another device. Work practices at the Dutch telemedical centre showed how telenurses could ignore frequent warnings of the telemonitoring system informing them that patients did not keep to the limits for weight and blood pressure, because they could rely on the phone. Telenurses used the phone to negotiate a change of the set standards with the polyclinic in order to eliminate these frequent reminders, particularly in cases where patients were not inclined to change their lifestyle. Dutch telenurses also relied on phone contacts with patients to reject a part of the script of the electronic triage system, which produced urgency scores: telenurses did not use them because they considered these assessments as not relevant to the health condition of chronic heart patients.

Work practices at the German telemedical centre showed similar examples of work-arounds. Telecare workers sometimes did not use the part of the script of the telemonitoring system that enabled them to assess ECGs. Instead they relied on phone contacts with patients because the phone enabled them to assess their heart problems using the contextual, situated knowledge of patients.

In Germany and the Netherlands, the phone thus turned out to be a useful technological device to work around part of the scripts of the other devices. The phone could be used in this way partly because of the flexible script of this technical device, and partly because of its weak alignment with the scripts of the other technological devices. Although the phone was meant to be used as a technology to support the other technological devices, that is, to gain access to information provided by patients, telecare workers used the phone as well to escape part of the scripts of the telemonitoring systems and the electronic triage system. Most importantly, the phone enables telecare workers to work around the abstract rationality inscribed in these digital systems. The use of the phone enabled them to build on and extend their practical knowledge. My analysis shows how telecare workers continue to value their own expertise and tacit knowledge: they do not passively follow the actions scripted in the digital devices but rely on their practical knowledge.

In addition to technological devices, telecare work is also shaped by labour politics. The German telemedical centre reflected demographic policies by locating its telemedical centre in the former East Germany and hiring 'Ossies' as telenurses and 'Wessies' as managers. The geography of telecare also reflects gender politics in which technical devices play an important role. In Germany and the Netherlands, telenurses' work is a female profession. As we have seen, the German telemedical centre explicitly selected women as telenurses because the management considered them better equipped for this work, relying on stereotypical images of feminine qualities. By employing women as telenurses and men as telephysicians and supervisors, the German centre, and to a lesser extent the Dutch centre, built on and reinforced the gendered hierarchy of labour that still dominates the healthcare sector in many countries. Work practices in the German centre indicate that women's telenursing work is more dependent on technological devices then men's work. As we have seen, telenurses do the actual work of operating the technical devices involved in delivering care remotely. Consequently, their work is directly shaped by the scripts of the technological devices. Although telephysicians' work also depends on technology, they work literally more at a distance from the devices. Whereas telenurse are bound to one specific location, that is, their computer desks, telephysicians can move around freely. Even more importantly, telephysicians' work is less structured by the scripts of the technological devices. In Germany, this flexibility is facilitated by a three-party-conference system incorporated in the phone, which enables them to escape the pre-structured actions inscribed in the telemonitoring system. Compared to the Dutch tele-medical centre, the German centre also delegates more flexibility and responsibility to telenurses because they do not have to use an electronic triage system to guide the phone-mediated interactions with patients.

Finally, telecare work is also defined by boundary work. As we have seen, the boundary work of traditional healthcare professionals resulted in a situation in which telecare work became restricted to advisory work. Medical interventions, that is, changing medication and producing diagnoses, remained in the hands of cardiologists, general practitioners, and heart-failure nurses. Telecare workers are expected to provide services to and support the work of traditional healthcare practitioners. The emerging landscape of telecare thus involves a distribution of labour based on the hierarchical relationship between telecare and traditional healthcare professionals. Work practices at the German telemedical centre indicate, however, that telephysicians do not always accept their restricted agency because they make (preliminary) diagnoses, particularly in the case of emergencies. Telephysicians, often supported by traditional healthcare practitioners, thus bypass the agreed division of labour.

Although practices at the telemedical centre suggest otherwise, telecare workers are formally and legally defined as proxies of traditional healthcare professionals. Based on my analysis, I conclude that a portrayal in terms of proxies is insufficient to describe the actual work performed by this new category of healthcare workers. The term 'proxies' suggests that telecare workers work only for traditional healthcare professionals who delegate specific tasks to them. By portraying telecare workers as proxies, dominant discourses intend to fix their position in the social and legal hierarchy of healthcare. As Mort and colleagues have described for nurses in a teledermatological clinic in the UK, nurses do much more than act as the proxies of doctors. Nurses often perform 'constitutive work' by filling in the gaps of knowledge created by the reductionist approach to healthcare inscribed in telecare technologies (Mort et al., 2003). My analysis shows a similar dynamic in which telenurses use their experiential and tacit knowledge to counterbalance the abstract and practical rationality required to provide healthcare remotely. Equally importantly, the proxy identity ascribed to telecare workers does not capture the role of technologies in defining this profession. Telecare workers should be considered as proxies not only of doctors but also of technologies. But even then telecare workers cannot be portrayed as proxies because this term suggests a technologically determinist view of telecare work. As I have described above, telecare workers do not passively follow the scripts of technological devices but actively develop work-arounds, which suggests a reciprocal relationship between telecare workers and technologies.

Following Mort, I therefore suggest that the kind of healthcare professionals created in the changing landscape of care can best be characterized as intermediary professionals. In contrast to the term 'proxies', which fixes telecare work in the social and legal hierarchy in healthcare, 'the role of intermediary is more fluid and hence challenging, widening the distribution of agency and the ownership of knowledge production' (Mort et al., 2003, p. 292). This discussion of the proxy identity ascribed to telecare workers is not only of academic relevance. Considering telecare professionals as proxies implies that most of their work remains invisible. Acknowledging them as intermediaries in healthcare may facilitate a process of professionalization in which telecare workers gain their own professional identity and become acknowledged as a separate specialist profession (Mort, 2003; Wahlberg, 2003).

Telecare workers can be considered intermediaries in a double sense. First, they act as intermediaries between technologies and patients. This intermediary work includes collecting information from patients, assessing patients' health condition based on biodata provided by tele-monitoring devices and their own experiential knowledge, instructing patients how to use the telemonitoring devices, and entering data in the electronic data systems. This kind of work clearly shows how telecare workers operate independently of traditional healthcare professionals and should be considered as professionals in their own right, not just as proxies of doctors. Second, telecare workers act as intermediaries between technologies, patients, and traditional healthcare profession-als. This intermediary work includes informing healthcare professionals about the results of telemonitoring, that is, the assessment of ECGs, weight or blood pressure, and contacting them to ask for medical interventions, such as changing medication or requiring admission to hospital. Although this kind of work reflects a hierarchy (telecare work-ers are not allowed to perform certain medical tasks), the agency and responsibility to initiate medical interventions is clearly delegated to telecare workers, assisted by telecare technologies.

Of course, this kind of intermediary work is not restricted to telecare workers. Similar work is performed by the assistants of general practi-tioners or by nurses in hospitals. One major difference, however, is that telecare workers have to do this intermediary work in the absence of patients. They do not see or get to know them personally because their interaction with patients is mediated by technological devices. The way in which telecare workers cope with the invisible patients is discussed in the following chapter.

6
How Places Matter in Healthcare: Physical and Digital Proximity

> Our proximity to or distance from others and from places has meaning for us.
>
> (Malone, 2003, p. 2317)

Since the late nineteenth century patients have become accustomed to visiting hospitals or the general practitioner when they are in need of care. For chronic patients these visits have become part and parcel of their life; because there is no cure for their diseases, they depend on regular consultations with healthcare professionals to adjust medical therapy to the progress of their illness.

Telecare technologies promise to change this form of healthcare by providing care remotely. Patients will not have to bother to visit the hospital but will be able to receive care very comfortably – or so it seems – at home. As described in Chapter 3, producers of telecare technologies also articulate other promises, that is, that telecare technologies will make healthcare more cost-effective and efficient. This promise can be realized only when current healthcare based on physical consultations is partly replaced by telecare encounters. This replacement policy is based on the implicit assumption that face-to-face care and telecare are basically the same. The means by which healthcare is delivered may change, but the content of healthcare will remain untouched. Telecare technologies are thus portrayed as tools that facilitate the delivery of healthcare. As I argued in Chapter 2, this rhetoric of delivery is problematic because it reinforces the image of technology as isolated instruments that can be inserted into healthcare without changing what care is all about. As sociologists of science, technology, and medicine have argued, technologies are not merely facilitators of care but should be considered as active transformers of healthcare

(Berg and Mol, 1998; Webster, 2002; Mol, 2002 and 2008). Instead of facilitating care, technologies interact with and shape the ways in which bodies and disorders are defined, treated, and experienced. The introduction of technologies such as diagnostic tools, protocols, and drugs creates differences and a multiplicity of treatments, bodies, patients and diseases rather than a coherent unity in which one technology smoothly replaces and replicates the other (Berg and Mol, 1998; Mol, 2002). We may thus expect telecare technologies to introduce differences into the existing kinds of care.

To analyse the different forms of care that emerge in face-to-face healthcare and telecare, I compare the healthcare provisions provided by nurses at policlinics for heart-failure patients with the emerging forms of care offered to these patients by nurses at a telemedical centre in the Netherlands. Since the mid-1990s, major hospitals in the Netherlands have established special outpatient departments known as heart-failure policlinics, staffed by the newly established nursing specialty of heart-failure nurses. In 2006 some of these policlinics participated in a clinical trial to test a telemonitoring system for heart-failure patients, The trial was initiated and financed by Achmea, a major Dutch health-insurance company and the medical division of Philips, one of the world's largest electronics companies. The testing of this new technology in cooperation with heart-failure policlinics enabled me to make a close comparison between these places in which acts of care take place. Drawing on the techno-geographical approach discussed earlier, the chapter aims to explore what it means when healthcare moves from physical to virtual spaces. How important are the places, which enable face-to-face contacts between doctors and patients? What forms of care are constituted in the polyclinics and new spaces of telemedical centres? This chapter begins with a discussion of studies on the changing spatial dimensions of healthcare, followed by an analysis of the healthcare provided in policlinics and telemedical centres. I argue that places matter in healthcare by describing how these spaces constitute different kinds of care that incorporate various definitions of nursing and illness.

Technologies and nurses' proximity to patients

In my analysis, I draw on insights developed by scholars in the field of human geography who are interested in the spatial dynamics of human relationships in healthcare. As Ruth Malone has suggested, being close to patients has been considered one of the key features of nursing. She defines nursing as 'a human practice to which relationship is considered essential'. Therefore nursing depends upon 'sustaining an often taken-for-granted proximity to patients' (Malone 2003, p. 2317). These traditional forms of proximity are drastically challenged by telecare technologies because they separate the nurse from the patient. Telecare technologies replace face-to-face contacts between nurses and patients with contacts mediated by telephone, television, webcam, and/or electronic networks. The absence of physical contact scripted in these technologies introduces a lack of vision and touch (for phone – and computer-based systems) and touch (for TV – and webcam-based systems). Studies of telecare therefore emphasize the consequences of the fact that nurses or physicians cannot see or touch patients. Because nurses are usually trained to make decisions based on observing patients, the absence of visual cues or the ability to touch the patient reduces the sources of information nurses can rely on, such as colour and texture of skin, odour, and body language (Johnson-Mekota et al., 2001, p. 32; Johnson Pettinari and Jessopp, 2001, p. 669; Wahlberg et al., 2003, p. 43; Mort et al., 2003). Studies of telephone-based health-advice provisions indicate that the inability to observe visible signs of illness influences the assessment of the patients' health condition and credibility (Johnson Pettinari and Jessopp, 2001, p. 670; Wahlberg et al., 2003). The challenge to nurses, particularly but not exclusively those working in telephone-based healthcare services, is that they must learn to rely on auditory rather than visual cues to know what is wrong with patients. Practices of 'seeing the patient' are replaced with practices of carefully listening to patients, both to what patients say and to auditory, non-verbal cues such as the degree of breath control and silences (Edwards, 1994). These studies thus suggest that the places in which acts of care take place matter. Physical spaces such as policlinics enable healthcare professionals to rely on resources other than telemedical centres to provide care.

In order to analyse the different forms of care created in policlinics and telemedical centres, I use the different forms of proximity introduced by Ruth Malone. In her study of the spatial dimensions of nurse–patient relationships, Malone described the different kinds of proximity that are threatened in current healthcare practices: physical, narrative, and moral proximity.[1] Physical proximity refers to 'a nearness within which nurses physically touch and care for patients' bodies (Malone, 2003, p. 2318). Narrative proximity is used to refer to practices in which 'nurses come to "know the patient" by hearing and trying to understand the patient's story' (Malone, 2003, p. 2318). Healthcare provisions introduced to monitor patients, both face-to-face and remote, change the nurses' traditional proximity to patients. Monitoring the health condition of so-called outpatients (patients discharged from hospital who still receive care) is delegated to nurses in polyclinics or telemedical centres that take over the care when patients leave the hospital. Telecare provisions clearly eliminate physical proximity, but physical proximity is challenged as well in face-to-face care because nurses in policlinics see the patient less frequently than in the hospital. Narrative proximity can be enacted in face-to-face as well as virtual encounters, but will be enacted in different ways. To capture the changes related to the introduction of telecare services, it is useful to distinguish yet another form of proximity: digital proximity, or proximity mediated by information and communication technologies. The question thus becomes: what kinds of care are created and valued or neglected in monitoring services based on physical or digital proximity to patients? What gets lost and what is gained when doctor–patient interactions move from physical to virtual encounters?

Physical proximity and care at the policlinic

'Eyes can tell you more': The importance of face-to-face contacts

Polyclinics that specialized in delivering care to chronic heart-failure patients discharged from hospital but still in need of care were established in the mid-1990s. These clinics can thus be considered as a rather recent innovation in healthcare. As telecare technologies, heart-failure policlinics are expected to lead to a decrease in the number and the length of hospital (re)admissions, thus reducing the costs of healthcare (Montfoort and Helm, 2006, p. 33; Chetney, 2003, p. 680).[2] The close monitoring of patients by specialized nurses in heart-failure policlynics or nurses in telemedical centres aims to help patients adhere to a bodily regime (including medication, diet and exercises) to reduce the risk of medical crises. Most heart-failure patients can be treated with a combination of drugs, diet, and lifestyle changes. However, in cases of late diagnosis, insufficient treatment, or non-compliance with therapy, the disorder can eventually be fatal (Montfort and Helm, 2006, p. 33). Early detection of worsening heart failure and its cause may prevent immediate transportation by ambulance to the hospital and admission to the emergency room (Cleland et al., 2005, p. 1654; Anonymous, 2004, p. 17).

The heart-failure policlinic investigated in this study was founded in 2001 by Medical Spectrum Twente (MST), the main general hospital in

Enschede in the Netherlands. Currently, all major Dutch hospitals run a heart-failure policlinic as part of their regular healthcare provisions. The emergence of heart-failure policlinics coincided with the rise of a new specialty in nursing: heart-failure nursing (Anonymous, 2004, p. 8, 9). In most Dutch academic and general hospitals, care traditionally given by cardiologists has been partly delegated to this new category of nurses. In the past decade, heart-failure nursing has developed into a profession with a high degree of autonomy in which nurses can advise, educate, supervise, diagnose, and treat heart-failure patients (Anonymous, 2004, p. 10). Currently, the heart-failure policlinic at the MST hospital provides care to approximately 650 patients. These include elderly but also younger patients, and is run by three qualified nurses assisted by a research physician and supervised by a cardiologist (Interview heart-failure nurse A, 2006). Heart-failure patients are referred to the policlinic when they are discharged from hospital, particularly those suffering from asthma cardiale: severe breathing problems caused by an impairment of the heart's pump function which results in redundant fluid that impairs the expansion of the lungs.

A first consultation at the policlinic consists of anamnesis (a short history of the development of the disease), explanation of the disease, measurement of blood pressure and weight,[3] advice concerning a healthy lifestyle, and the prescription of medication. Follow-up consultations consist of monitoring the health condition of patients and their compliance with medication and the bodily regime (Inspectie Gezondheidszorg, 2003, p. 14). To perform the multiple tasks involved in a consultation in the policlinic, nurses can rely on various resources to assess the conditions of patients, including an electronic database, measurement of weight and blood pressure, laboratory tests, and observation of the patient. Of these different resources, observations are considered crucial. Nurses at the policlinic emphasized the importance of 'seeing the patient'. As one nurse put it:

> The looks of a patient can tell you how they are doing ... I want to see how tight in the chest he is, how swollen his legs or how blue his hands or lips are. I want to see it.
>
> (Interview heart-failure nurse A, 2006)

As has been described for other nurses (Johnson-Mekota et al., 2001; Johnson Pettinari and Jessop, 2001), heart-failure nurses in the policlinic experience nursing as a profession with a visual attitude, although listening to patients, particularly to detect shortness of breath, is also considered important. In the stories nurses told us, they easily switched between visual and auditory cues as important elements in their assessment:

Nurses are very much attuned to vision. This is what you learn in your training: 'are there changes, do you notice anything when you look at the patient? Does he have swollen feet? Is he short of breath?' You listen to the patient. You just look at the patient.

(Interview heart-failure nurse C, 2006)

Although auditory resources thus play a role in the evaluation of patients' accounts of their illness, nurses prioritize visual cues. According to nurses, patients may often tell them they are doing fine, even when they have swollen feet or breathing problems:

Sometimes patients do not tell you what is wrong, simply because they do not want to be ill ... In the policlinic I can see them. Maybe very simple, but this is how it is.

(Interview heart-failure nurse C, 2006)

Visual resources are considered as even more important than the objective measurement of blood pressure:

Look, blood pressure tells you a lot, but not everything. Someone can have a nice blood pressure but look very miserable. Blood pressure does not reveal that. Therefore you want to keep seeing your patients. Eyes can always tell you more than

(Interview heart-failure nurse B, 2006)

Visual cues are thus more valued than other resources, particularly when nurses detect contradictions in the measurements of bodily indicators or the accounts of patients (Interview heart-failure nurses B and C, 2006).

The 'crying policlinic': Knowing the patient and psychosocial care

Physical proximity to patients at the heart-failure policlinic is important not only to monitor the physical condition of patients but also in other respects. First, physical nearness enables nurses to communicate with patients with hearing deficiencies or patients who do not speak Dutch, particularly elderly immigrants from Turkey and Morocco. In face-to-face contacts with these patients, nurses can rely on non-verbal communication, or 'talking with your hands and feet' (Interview heart-failure nurse B, 2006). Physical encounters at the heart-failure clinic also enable recently migrated patients to invite an interpreter, often a close relative, to accompany him or her to the consultation (Interview heart-failure nurse B, 2006).

Second, physical proximity enables nurses to build a relationship with patients, or, as one nurse put it:

> I simply realised that a tie arises between patients and us as heart-failure nurses. It is definitely different than at the cardiology department in the hospital. You have much more time for people. People trust you very much.
>
> (Interview heart-failure nurse C, 2006)

These close relationships between nurses and patients play an important role in lowering the threshold for patients to call nurses in case they gain weight or experience breathing problems. This is important because, as described above, an early detection of the problem may prevent immediate hospitalization (Interview Balk, 2005). Knowing patients personally also plays an important role in learning to interpret patients' accounts of their illness. Because of the wide variety of complaints that patients voice their complaints – ranging from exaggerating to underestimating heart-failure symptoms – nurses have to rely on their knowledge of a patient's character to decide how they should evaluate a patient's story.

As with nurses, cardiologists also consider it as crucial to 'know the patient', not only to interpret the ways in which complaints are voiced but also to differentiate between the various ways in which heart-failure symptoms are expressed, and they value this more than seeing the patient over a longer period of time:

> If I have seen the patient several times, and I know the patient, then you can tell 'this is the weak spot of the patient'. If you know patients then you can tell that if they are not doing well they do not eat anymore. Another patient will be more short of breath. If you know these nuances of patients I can tell by phone, without seeing him, that he should visit the clinic.
>
> (Interview Balk, 2006)

Coming to know the patient thus seems to take place particularly during face-to-face contacts at the beginning of the care trajectory.

If relationships with patients are well established, 'seeing the patient' becomes less important and a first assessment of the seriousness of patients' complaints can be done by phone. What all these experiences indicate is that physical proximity enables nurses to come to know the patient as a person as well as his or her illness. This is in line with Malone's argument that physical proximity is important to create narrative proximity, a term she introduced to refer to processes in which nurses come to 'know the patient' by hearing and trying to understand the patient's story (Malone, 2003, p. 2318). Narrative proximity can thus be considered as an important aspect of nursing at the heart-failure policlinic and is crucial for the kind of care provided at this clinic.

Finally, physical proximity enables nurses to help patients cope with the disease. The diagnosis of heart failure has severe consequences for patients. They not only have to change their lifestyle and diet, take their medicines regularly, and measure their weight and blood pressure daily; they also have to learn to come to terms with the fatal consequences of the disease. Learning to cope with the disease may involve intensive psychosocial stress for which patients are often unable to find adequate support in their own environment. Therefore, heart-failure clinics consider the provision of psychosocial support as central to the care they give to patients. Actually, psychosocial care can be considered one of the major achievements of heart-failure policlinics. Prior to the existence of these outpatients' departments, care for heart-failure patients was restricted to medical care (Interview heart-failure nurse A, 2006). Psychosocial care is provided not only to patients but also to their close relatives. Close relatives, often the patient's partner, are explicitly invited to accompany patients to consultations at the heart-failure policlinic. Nurses thus have to deal with the emotions of patients and their partners. Consultations at the heart-failure policlinic often involve expressions of strong emotions and a lot of crying. Consequently, the heart-failure policlinic is often referred to as the 'crying policlinic' (Interview heart-failure nurse A, 2006). Psychosocial care is provided not only at the policlinic; nurses also organize thematic afternoons and refer patients and their partners, often separately, to social workers at the hospital (Interview heart-failure nurse A, 2006). Contacts with partners of patients also provide nurses with an extra resource for coming to know what the illness means in daily life for the patient and his or her family, including problems related to compliance with the bodily regime and medication. Patients' partners are thus crucial to realizing the two aspects of narrative proximity described by

Malone: they inform nurses about the illness of the patient; and, vice versa, nurses can transmit their knowledge to 'others', in this case the partners who care for patients. Actually, heart-failure nurses even go one step further. They not only transmit their knowledge to partners, but also invite them to play an active role in caring for patients, particularly to help male patients maintain their diet. Nurses thus enrol partners as important intermediaries to extend their span of control over patients' compliance with the patients' home. Like the provision of psychosocial care, the involvement of partners in care is one of the major achievements of the heart-failure policlinic.

We can conclude that the physical proximity to patients created in the policlinic facilitates contextualized and personalized care: patients are approached as part of a relational setting and care plans are attuned to the character and lifestyle of the patients. In this form of care, nurses act as counsellors of patients and have a high degree of autonomy. Responsibilities for monitoring, including diagnosis, supervision, and treatment, are delegated primarily to nurses.

Digital proximity and care at telemedical centres

Building relationships with patients: The importance of phone contacts

Like heart-failure policlinics, telemedical centres are a rather recent innovation in the delivery of healthcare to chronic patients. The telemedical centre investigated in this study, the Medical Service Centre, was established in 2002 by Achmea, one of the major health-insurance companies in the Netherlands. As described in the previous chapter, the telecare services provided by this centre include a health-advice line; health assistance during holidays ('the holiday doctor'), and the coordination of transport services to hospitals (Interview Boutkan and Helm, 2006). All these services are based on a computer-assisted triage system run by 50, often part-time, employees (Interview Sorgdrager and Borst 2006). In 2006, the health insurance company decided to collaborate with Philips to test the heart-failure telemonitoring system developed by this firm in the insurer's telemedical centre. In January 2008, the health insurance company included the telemonitoring service for heart-failure patients they had tested in previous years in accordance with their basic insurance policy. This means that heart-failure patients insured by this company can receive this form of care at no additional cost (Zilveren Kruis/Achmea, 2008).

The decision to include the Achmea Medical Service Centre as an intermediary infrastructure in the testing and implementation of the heart-failure telemonitoring system in the Netherlands was a second choice. Initially, Philips tried to use a telemedical centre in Germany to facilitate the implementation of its new technology simultaneously in Germany and the Netherlands. Owing to resistance from Dutch cardiologists, Philips had to withdraw this plan and opted for the Dutch telemedical centre (Interview Balk, 2006). The resistance of Dutch cardiologists to a telemedical centre in Germany illustrates how places where healthcare takes place matter, not only in terms of how spaces shape proximity to patients, which is the major focus of this chapter, but also in terms of the physical, geographical context of healthcare. Although in principle telemedical centres can be located anywhere because they deliver healthcare remotely, the places where telemedical centres are positioned remain important for healthcare. In this respect, there seems to be an important difference between call centres for commercial purposes and call centres or telemedical centres that provide healthcare services. Whereas commercial call centres are often located in other countries than their customers (usually cheap labour countries in Asia), healthcare cannot be so easily turned into a global, locally unbounded commodity. One of the reasons is differences in language, which is considered as a major barrier to providing healthcare. Dutch cardiologists involved in heart-failure telecare, as well as Dutch general practitioners affiliated with the Hartis Medical Service Centre which provides telecare for heart rhythm patients, emphasized the importance of language. In their view, calls of Dutch patients to a telemedical centre should be answered by Dutch native speakers to set patients' minds at ease and to build trusting relationships with patients (Interview Balk 2005, interview Jurgens, 2004). The resistance to German-speaking telecare workers also illustrates how the history of World War II still shapes the relationships between German and Dutch citizens, particularly elderly patients, who associate German with the language of the German occupiers in the period 1940–45. Consequently, telemedical centres cannot be located just anywhere, particularly not in Germany.

After this short detour, let me return again to the analysis of care provided at the Achmea Medical Service Centre in Zwolle. Telecare provided at telemedical centres involves a major change in nurses' proximity to patients. Whereas heart-failure nurses in the policlinic interact with patients face-to-face, telenurses rely on computer- and phone-mediated contacts. Instead of open communication initiated by nurses or patients, nurse–patient interactions at the telemedical centre are guided by the telemonitoring system, an electronic triage system (TAS), and a telephone. Physical proximity is thus replaced by contacts mediated by new and old media technologies. As described in the previous chapter, the new media technologies in particular provide nurses with a strict regime of nurse–patient interactions. The telemonitoring system urges nurses to watch their computer screen regularly to notice warnings deviations in patients' weight or blood pressure and call patients as soon as a warning is detected. Telenurses are also expected to phone the patient to enquire about the cause of their increased weight or blood pressure or to call the heart-failure policlinic to change medication required to stabilize blood pressure or reduce weight. As we have seen, the actions scripted in the technological devices leave almost no room for the responsibility, expertise, and tacit knowledge of nurses. Consequently, telecare work is constituted as highly pre-structured and protocol-driven work. However, my analysis of the practices in the Achmea telemedical centre showed that telenurses ignore the protocols inscribed in the technology but develop work-arounds to provide care that meets their own standards. This also happens in the way telenurses interact with patients, in which the phone emerges again as an important tool.

Like heart-failure nurses, telenurses consider 'knowing the patient' an important aspect of providing care. From interviews with nurses at the telemedical centre we learned that the frequency of phone contacts is an important condition to create relationships of trust with patients. As with physical proximity, digital proximity has a temporal dimension that depends on a minimum of contacts to create the nearness to patients required to provide proper care. Because nurse–patient relationships cannot be established in face-to-face contacts, the temporal dimension becomes more consequential. As described in the previous chapter, the script of the telemonitoring system allows nurses to contact patients only in case of deviating weight or blood pressure. Consequently, the frequency of contacts with patients who do not exceed the set limits will be very low. Nurses consider the restrictions on phone contacts scripted in the technology as the most difficult aspect of telemonitoring, or as one nurse put it:

> When patients are not doing well, you may have daily contacts for a certain period. But with people who are doing fine, you may have contact only once in four months. This is the difficult side of telemonitoring: it is not so much the technical aspects, or the interpretative work, but to gain patients' confidence.
>
> (Interview Sorgdrager, 2006)

The team leader of the telenurses articulated similar concerns and emphasized the ambivalence created by the technology:

> This is the difficulty with our role in telemonitoring. On the one hand, we would like to have contacts with patients; on the other hand, we notice that there is less need for contacts because of the telemonitoring system. Our experiences with the diversity among patients is that some patients prefer to have frequent contacts whereas others would like to have less contact. It is very hard to find the right balance.
>
> (Interview Wal, 2006)

To meet their own standards of care, telenurses established a practice in which they overruled the script of the technology or, as the physician told us:

> In the beginning we did not call without any reason. When there was no medical indication, we did not call and we could not build a relationship. We take more initiatives now and then you learn that there is a willingness. But it takes time and you will have to find a good modus for each patient.
>
> (Interview Borst, 2006)

Telecare workers thus prioritized their own experiential knowledge over the rules prescribed by the telemonitoring system. In their view, the technology had taken over too much of their responsibility. Because nurses are trained to grasp the whole situation before deciding on the care they can give, they wanted to keep the initiative to contact patients in their own hands instead of delegating this to the technology (Interview Sorgdrager and Borst, 2006). For telecare workers the frequency of contact is thus important not only in building trusting relationships with patients but also for gaining control over the care they give.

'Your ears become your eyes': Assessing physical changes

As described above, the most important difference between nurse–patient interactions in the policlinic and the telemedical centre is that telenurses can only phone patients whereas heart-failure nurses can communicate both by phone and face to face. For telenurses it took some time to become accustomed to the absence of visual resources. As the telephysician explained:

> Not seeing is the big difference. In the beginning we had to get used to it very much. You are used to make your diagnosis or create an

understanding through a combination of what you hear and body language. Sometimes this does not match. Also, someone can look pale or is sweaty; these kind of things are left out when you work with telephone contact only.

(Interview Borst, 2006)

Colour or moisture of skin and body language are thus considered as important visual cues that are absent as resources for telenurses' work. Because of the lack of visual resources, active listening has become a crucial skill to assess the health condition of patients. Or, as Johnson Pettinari and Jessop (2001, p. 672) sum up the nurses' work at health-advice lines: 'Your ears become your eyes.' A similar practice has been established at the telemedical centre. All nurses have received training to become acquainted with phone communication and have developed specific skills for active listening in their previous work for other telecare provisions at the centre. To quote the telephysician:

The ear is just as important as the voice. During my work at the doctor's advice line we have learned a completely different way of listening. We are very much used to listening, to listening between the lines, that is what we have developed. And it really works, maybe even more than for someone who is used to seeing people and only lifts the phone once in a while. You can hear the breathing, the surrounding environment, the anxiety of the people nearby, or the partner. These things also tell you something.

(Interview Borst, 2006)

To make up for the lack of visual cues, telecare workers depend not only on listening skills but also on communicative skills. For the physical indications of poor health they cannot see, nurses will ask specific questions such as the color of skin, whether patients feel tired, or whether they are sweating. Or, as the physician told us: 'What I cannot see, I have to ask [about]' (Interview Borst, 2006).[4] Communication skills are very important to providing care to heart-failure patients, not only because nurses cannot see the patients but also because they constitute a difficult category of patients. Because of the chronic nature of their illness, the symptoms of heart failure are often more subtle than for acute diseases. Moreover, patients have become used to living with some pain, or with being tired, or with having swollen legs once in a while. Learning to keep asking questions is thus an important skill that requires intensive training and learning by doing. Usually it takes several months before telenurses have acquired this skill (Interview Borst and Wal, 2006). Communication skills are thus crucial resources in providing care at a distance. In the end, however, telenurses rely very much on their intuition:

> You can never switch off your what we call 'wrong-not wrong' feeling. That is a sixth sense that you have and in which you have to learn to have confidence. If you have developed this, then you learn to trust it and you do not deny it. Even if someone gives only negative answers to all your questions and the TAS-system remains white [no score of urgency]: at the moment that your sixth sense tells you 'something is not right', you have to act accordingly.
>
> (Interview Borst, 2006)

Equally importantly, telenurses have learned to accept the boundaries of the care they can provide. In situations where the physician thinks it is important to do physical examinations such as using a stethoscope, they will refer the patient to another healthcare professional. Knowing when to refer to other healthcare providers is considered an important expertise of telecare workers (Interview Borst, 2006).

From obstacle to provision of equal care: The advantage of not 'seeing the patient'

Based on their training and experience, healthcare professionals at the telemedical centre have learned to consider the absence of face-to-face contacts with patients as a challenge rather than something 'scary', a feeling they initially had (Interview Borst, 2006). In the interviews they emphasized that there are also advantages when you do not have face-to-face contacts with patients. Because of someone's appearance, nurses are often inclined to create a certain image of the patients' personality and health condition or, as the physician put it:

> The advantage is that you will treat each patient the same way because you do not have any prejudice, you do not think: 'Oh, what a theatrical person'.
>
> (Interview Borst, 2006)

The absence of visual cues thus prevents telecare workers from making hasty judgements based on visual features alone. Most crucially, not seeing the patient is transformed from an obstacle to providing proper care into a condition that facilitates equal care for all patients, independent of their appearance. These experiences of telecare workers thus reveal an ambivalent view of vision. On the one hand, telecare workers consider visual cues as relevant resources to assess the health condition of patients, and have to put in quite some effort to make up for the absence of visual resources. On the other hand, telecare workers experience seeing the patient as a disadvantage because their judgements of the patient's appearance add a constraint to giving adequate care. The interviews with telecare workers thus indicate that they have developed skills to deal with and carefully balance the perceived disadvantages and advantages of the absence of physical proximity.

The experiences of telenurses also show an important difference in narrative proximity in the telemedical centre as compared with the heart-failure policlinic. Whereas heart-failure nurses constructed their assessment of patients' conditions from various bodily indicators and patients' and their partners' stories about the illness, telenurses rely on a more limited set of medical indicators (only weight and blood pressure and no lab tests) and patients' answers to the pre-structured questions of the TAS system that, however, do not include psychosocial accounts. The narrative proximity created at the telemedical centre is thus more focused on bodily indicators of the patients' health. Moreover, the use of pre-structured questions reduces the chance of proximity rather than encouraging it. Reflecting on the second aspect of narrative proximity as described by Malone, that is, how nurses transmit their knowledge to others; the telemedical centre also shows a different picture than the heart-failure policlinic. Instead of transferring knowledge to patients and their partners, the telemedical centre transfers knowledge primarily to patients. Graphs of weight and blood pressure, videos to explain the illness or give advice on diet, and overviews of medication are sent to the patient at home. Although partners or other family members or inhabitants can look at the data too,[5] if the patient allows this, the graphs are meant to serve as tools to provide self-care. Although others can give support to patients' self-care, they are not actively enrolled in providing or supporting care. Digital proximity thus creates a narrative proximity in which partners, or others who care for patients, are not included or made responsible.

On the other hand, digital proximity facilitates a form of care that provides patients with systematic tools for self-care, a resource that is not available to patients who receive care in the heart-failure policlinic. Although heart-failure nurses also encourage patients to take care of their health, the telemonitoring system transforms self-care into an obligation. If telenurses do not receive the patients' daily measurements of weight and blood pressure, they will remind patients to provide them. Telemonitoring technology thus drastically changes healthcare for heart-failure patients because it introduces a daily surveillance of patients' health condition that enables experts to monitor patients' self-care. Whereas care provided by the heart-failure policlinic is characterized by monitoring the health condition of patients in regular time interludes, the telemedical centre provides a form of care in which monitoring is transformed into a continuous process. The increased temporal nearness to patients facilitates a form of care in which patients receive immediate care (medication or hospital admission) in the case of a medical crisis.

In summary, the digital proximity created at the telemedical centre introduces an individualized, immediate form of care that makes self-care an obligation. In this form of care, nurses act as surveillants. Moreover, they are granted much less autonomy than nurses at the policlinic. As I described in the previous chapter, the telemonitoring system provides nurses with a strict regime of nurse–patient interactions in which the responsibility to detect changes in patients' physical condition is delegated to the technology. Moreover, the responsibility for changing medication is delegated to healthcare professionals at the policlinic.

Conclusions

Based on the techno-geographical analysis presented in this chapter, I conclude that the places where healthcare occurs still matter. Despite representations of telecare technologies which suggest that healthcare can be turned into globally, locally unbounded practices, this chapter shows how the spaces in which acts of care take place shape what care is provided. Healthcare provided by the telemedical centre does not replicate the conventional healthcare provided at the heart-failure policlinics; it introduces a different kind of care. The major differences between these two forms of healthcare are summarized in table 6.1.

This overview clearly shows that the policlinic and the telemedical centre create and value different kinds of care, based on different forms of proximity to patients. The physical proximity created at the heart-failure clinic facilitates contextualized, personalized care in which open communication and dialogue with patients and their partners are valued as important aspects of medical and psychosocial care. The digital proximity that characterizes the telemedical centre supports individualized, immediate care in which protocol-driven communication, daily

Table 6.1   Different forms of care provided by policlinics and telemedical centres

Physical proximity	Digital proximity
intermittent monitoring	daily monitoring
open communication	protocol-driven communication
medical interventions and advice	control and advice
nurse as counsellor	nurse as surveillant
psychosocial care through dialogue	psychosocial care via video
self-care as option	self-care as obligation
‖	‖
V	V
contextualized, personalized care that constitutes heart-failure as illness	individualized, immediate care that constitutes heart-failure as disease

surveillance, and self-care emerge as important dimensions of care. Most importantly, neither form of healthcare leaves the established practices of nursing and medicine untouched. First, they actively intervene to shape the autonomy of nurses. In the policlinic, the responsibility for monitoring, including diagnosis, supervision and treatment is primarily delegated to nurses. Heart-failure nurses act as counsellors to patients and have a high degree of autonomy. In the telemedical centre nurses are granted much less autonomy. In this telemediated environment the responsibility for detecting changes in the health condition of patients is largely delegated to technical devices. Moreover, the responsibility for changing medication is delegated to healthcare professionals at the policlinic. Telenurses are expected to act primarily as surveillants who control the physical condition of patients based on the information provided by the telemonitoring technology and the electronic triage system. This chapter thus contributes to recent debates on autonomy and responsibilities in healthcare. Whereas other researchers have described how technologies shape the autonomy of patients (Lehoux et al., 2004), my study indicates that technology plays an active role in redefining the autonomy of nurses. The introduction of the telemonitoring technology for heart-failure patients implies that nurses are allowed to act only when the system has detected a deviation from the set standards for weight and blood pressure. My analysis shows how telenurses sometimes resist this form of nursing because they consider it important to have more contact with patients than the system allows in providing care that meets their own standards.

Second, the healthcare provided at the policlinic and the telemedical centre not only differ in terms of the autonomy granted to nurses, but also involve different definitions and treatments of heart-failure. The physical proximity to patients created in the policlinic facilitates open communication and enables nurses to know the patient as a person as well as his or her disorder. As we have seen, patients' and their partners' experiences and feelings play an important role in the monitoring of patients. Equally importantly, the care provided to patients is not restricted to medical care but also includes psychosocial care. Psychosocial care can be considered the major achievement of heart-failure policlinics compared to the conventional care provided by cardiologists. Drawing on the distinction between illness and disease commonly used in social studies of medicine (Mol, 2002, p. 9), in which illness refers to healthcare practices that include medical and psycho-social aspects and take into account patients' stories and experiences, whereas disease refers to practices in which the treatment of disorders relies only on medical expertise of healthcare professionals, I conclude that the care provided at the policlinic constitutes heart-failure as an illness. In contrast, the focus on the physical condition of patients and the expertise of healthcare professionals in the telemedical centre con-stitutes heart failure as a disease. The daily surveillance of bodily indi-cators assisting immediate medical care in case of crises can be viewed as the main asset of telecare services. However, the definition of heart failure as a disease also has disadvantages for patients because it neglects the psychosocial aspects or care. The choice of providing care based on either physical or digital proximity can thus be consequential for the ways in which disorders are defined and treated: as either illness or dis-ease. Equally importantly, patients may prefer the physical proximity to nurses at the policlinic over the digital proximity of telemedical centres. The ways in which patients relate to these two different forms of care are discussed in Chapter 8. The next chapter also addresses the inter-actions between patients and telecare technologies, but first addresses the work it takes to produce patients who are active and responsible as participants in the diagnosis of heart problems.

Part III
Redefining Patients and Home

7
Patients as Diagnostic Agents: Invisible Work and Selective Use

Telecare technologies drastically transform the order of who cares. As described in the first chapter, major parts of healthcare are delegated to patients. Instead of passive recipients, they are expected to become active and responsible participants in the diagnosis and monitoring of health disorders. In the changing landscape of healthcare, patients are thus configured as key actors. This active role of patients is, however, largely absent from the dominant discourses on telecare technologies. As we have seen in Chapter 3, the promises articulated on the websites of telecare companies are restricted to a description of the instrumental tasks involved in patients' use of telecare devices. By referring to actors and care practices in terms of healthcare providers and healthcare delivery, the promises suggest that telecare relies on an active sender (i.e., a healthcare professional) and a passive receiver (i.e., a patient), thus reinforcing the order of care in which only healthcare professionals do healthcare work. Drawing on the techno-geographical approach discussed earlier, I suggest that it is crucial to counter this image by making visible the actual work patients do in telecare practices. As described in the second chapter, a techno-geographical approach is a useful heuristic not only to study how places matter in healthcare but also to understand how technical devices delegate actions and responsibilities to people and technological objects. Whereas the previous chapters described how telecare technologies participate in changing the work practices and responsibilities of healthcare professionals, this chapter includes patients as major actors in the emerging landscape of telecare.

This chapter aims to make up for the absence of patients in dominant discourses on telecare by examining the use of ambulatory ECG recorders in the Netherlands. These portable devices for registering, recording and transmitting electrocardiograms (ECGs) have been developed to assist in the diagnosis and monitoring of irregularities of the heart rhythm across distances. For patients, the use of this telecare device is very consequential because it may involve a gradual transition from a healthy individual to a person at risk and eventually to a patient suffering from a specific (chronic) illness. Diagnostic technologies such as the ambulatory ECG recorder mediate and intervene in this process by providing the means to address the grey zone of doubt: Are my heart rate problems only temporary and within the range of normal heart functions, or do they indicate that something is seriously wrong? For many patients, the ambulatory ECG recorder can become the messenger that will change their identities from healthy individuals to heart patients. Telecare devices such as the ambulatory ECG recorder can thus be considered as 'disciplinary techniques performed by and upon bodies' (Cartwright, 2000, p. 354), tools that can facilitate or constrain this transition of identities.

Telecare technologies transform the diagnosis of heart rhythm disturbances because they open up, or close down, options and subjectivities, a process that Brown and Webster have described as a 'defining feature of the new digital and genetic technologies' (Brown and Webster, 2004, p. 51). The use of the ambulatory ECG recorder constitutes the subject as an alert and active individual who pays close attention to all possible changes in his or her heart rhythm and cooperates with healthcare professionals in speeding up the diagnosis. The technology invites patients to play an active role in their own diagnosis by delegating crucial parts of the work to patients. This may induce two different processes. On the one hand, it may increase the already existing anxiety (Do I have a serious heart disease? Do I have the skills to use this device? Can I trust this technology?), resulting in the selective use or non-use of the device. On the other hand, telecare technologies provide a tool with which to regain mastery of the circumstances. The ambulatory ECG recorder thus grants individuals a certain subjectivity and agency to make the passage from a healthy person to an individual suffering from a mild or serious illness. Options and subjectivities that are closed down by the technology include accepting or backgrounding irregularities of your heart rhythm and leaving the diagnostic work solely in the hands of the doctor.

The work delegated to patients thus goes far beyond the instrumental tasks described in the promises on telecare producers' patient websites. Patients are expected not only to use a technology but also to monitor their bodies and perform subjectivities related to bodily (in)competencies. We thus may wonder how and whether patients succeed in becoming active participants in the diagnosis of heart problems. To examine the work involved in this process, I draw on insights developed by scholars studying invisible work, particularly the late Leigh Star and the late Anselm Strauss. Star and Strauss introduced the concept of invisibility to help to understand the 'ecology of visible and invisible work' (Star and Strauss, 1999). In their study, invisibility refers to the neglect of representing specific knowledge and skills as formal work. They argued that the question of 'what counts as work' shapes the invisibility of specific expertise and specific groups of actors (Strauss, 1985; Star and Strauss, 1999). Although the people who perform this work are quite visible, the work they do is relegated to the background (Star and Strauss, 1999, p. 20). To capture the invisible work involved in making technologies work, Strauss and colleagues introduced the concept of articulation work, which refers to 'work that gets things back "on track" in the face of the unexpected, and modifies action to accommodate unanticipated contingencies' (Strauss, 1985). The study of articulation work has been central to the field of computer-supported cooperative work, where scholars argued that social scientists and designers should not restrict their analyses to 'production work' but should include 'the hidden task of articulation work' to aid understanding of why information systems work or do not work (Star, 1999, p. 387; Schmidt and Simone, 1996). As Leigh Star has suggested, all of us may perform articulation work to keep our work going (Star, 1999, p. 310). Most empirical studies of invisible work focus, however, on work in occupational contexts, except for feminist studies of housewives and Star's early work on parents (Cowan, 1983; Star, 1989). I suggest that it is important to extend the study of invisible work from occupational contexts to situations outside formal work relations, particularly the work of patients.[1] Following Strauss et al. (1997), my choice to describe the tasks and responsibilities delegated to patients by telecare technologies as work is an explicit strategy that is crucial in the techno-geographical approach developed in this book. By labelling their actions as work, I argue that healthcare work does not disappear because of telecare technologies, a view that is often articulated in dominant discourse but delegated to patients.

For analysing the articulation work involved in telecare technologies, Schmidt and Simone's definition is most useful. They describe articulation work as 'work that manages the consequences of the distributed nature of work' (Schmidt and Simone, 1996). Like the information systems designed to support collaborative work, telecare technologies can be characterized as network technologies that distribute healthcare work among various actors and locations. As described in the first chapter, the introduction of telecare technologies implies that more, geographically separated, actors will become involved in the work required to produce diagnoses. The diagnostic use of the ambulatory ECG recorder includes patients, home-care nurses, general practitioners' assistants, general practitioners, and telephysicians. In this emerging geography of care, all the actors will have to perform articulation work to manage the consequences of this distributed work.

In this chapter I examine the invisible work of patients as well as the work home-care nurses and telephysicians perform invisibly to assist patients to become active participants in the diagnosis of heart problems. I begin with an analysis of how patients try to master the new technology in their home environment and public spaces. The chapter proceeds with an examination of the work involved in instructing patients and the ways in which the telemedical centre assists them to play an active role in the diagnosis of their heart problems. The chapter concludes with a discussion of how we can understand that people who are anxious about their hearts can become active participants in healthcare.

Acting as diagnostic agents: The invisible work of patients at home

To understand the work delegated to patients, it is useful to start with the instruction card that patients receive when they first receive an ambulatory ECG-recorder. These instructions are very straightforward. The brief user manual, printed on a plastic card, includes five different actions. First, patients have to attach the ECG recorder, a small round box, to their bodies by sticking two electrodes on their chest by using special band-aids, inserting the plug of a small cable connected to the electrodes on the bottom of the recorder, and fixing the ECG recorder to their waist-band. When the recorder is properly fixed to the body, the patients have to produce an ECG-recording by pushing the 'record' button of the ECG recorder. When the patient has made four ECGs, the recorder gives a long beep signal telling the patient to submit the recorded ECGs to the telemedical centre via a regular or mobile phone. To do so, the patient has to remove the recorder from the waist band, dial the telephone number of the service centre, and wait for a connection and further instructions. When the staff at the telemedical centre answer the phone, they tell patients to send their ECGs. Patients then have to hold the telephone microphone firmly over the speaker at the front side of the recorder and push the 'send' button until they hear the beep sound that accompanies the sending of the ECGs. After sending the ECGs, patients have to delete the recordings by pushing the record button again. Finally, the patients have to maintain the ECG recorder and check the cable cords for splits or cracks (Instruction card Hartis).

Reflecting on these instructions, it is obvious that the user manual only includes instrumental tasks that rely on what Lehrer has called 'procedural' or 'practical knowledge' (Lehrer, 1990). Like the promises included in the telecare websites, the instructions thus give a very narrow view of the work and responsibilities delegated to patients. As described above, these instrumental tasks constitute only a minor part of the work patients have to do when the ambulatory ECG recorder enters their lives. To capture this invisible work of patients, I introduce the concept of the diagnostic agent: patients are not just users of a new technology that requires instrumental skills, but should be considered as agents who have to perform all manner of articulation work required to carry out the responsibilities delegated to them. In the new geography of responsibilities inscribed in the ambulatory ECG recorder, the most difficult task is delegated to patients: they are expected to catch the right moment to register an ECG that shows their heart rate dysfunction. Our interviews with patients indicate that many patients experienced it as difficult to decide when to register an ECG.[2] Selecting the right moment to make an ECG touches at the very heart of the new technology. As described in Chapter 3, the very aim of the ambulatory ECG recorder is to capture irregularities of the heart rhythm that occur very infrequently and unexpectedly. Making an ECG requires patients to pay close attention to their own heart rhythm and to assess the seriousness and nature of their heart problem. The ability to decide which irregularity is 'bad enough' to register and send requires a very specific type of knowledge that cannot be acquired by training. The only instructions the patients receive are to make an ECG whenever they feel their heart rate is irregular. The responsibility for selecting the right moment is thus delegated to patients without clear guidance. What counts as an irregularity worth registering is solely in the hands of patients: they have to decide by themselves without further assistance from medical professionals. Becoming a 'diagnostic agent' thus depends on a process of self-learning where patients have to trust their own ability to make the right choices.

This part of the work required to operate the new technology clearly illustrates how telecare devices shift responsibilities and agencies to patients. Work previously performed by cardiologists, general practitioners, or nurses is delegated to individuals with no previous experience or education in these matters. Problems in the diagnosis of heart rhythm irregularities that cannot be solved by other diagnostic devices are now delegated to the new diagnostic device and to patients.

Patients' experiences in making ECGs show that recording an irregular and infrequent dysfunction of the heartbeat is very difficult and demanding work that requires close self-monitoring of patients' own bodies. The reasons patients gave for why they considered it difficult to choose the right moment to make an ECG are manifold and varied. Some patients found it difficult to make ECGs at night:

> I have serious rhythm disturbances at night and I do not feel so well then. So I didn't make an ECG.
>
> (Woman, age 76)

Other patients faced problems because of the infrequency of their heart rate irregularities:

> The disturbances in my heart beat are very short and infrequent and therefore difficult to catch.
>
> (Woman, age 26)

Choosing the right moment to make an ECG turned out to be very complicated for patients who suffered from multiple illnesses:

> I have other complaints as well (gullet and stomach) and found it difficult to tell the difference.
>
> (Woman, age 53)

> Sometimes I was tired but did not know whether it was caused by my heart. I can be tired because I am short of breath as well.
>
> (Woman, age 81)

Other patients experienced problems making an ECG because they felt they were always too late:

> I always wondered for a moment, should I push the button now or should I wait a while. I did not want to push too quickly. I often thought: 'I will push the next time', but I only thought it and did not do it.
>
> (Woman, age 39)

Obviously, these patients were not informed sufficiently or had forgotten the instructions which explained that the ambulatory ECG recorder stores two minutes of the continuously recorded ECG before they push the 'record' button and one minute after they have activated the system. Finally, the poor health of some heart patients proved to be a major barrier to making ECGs:

> Sometimes I felt very weak and almost fainted. At such moments you do not think of the recorder at all. When it was over, I thought that pushing the button did not make sense anymore.
>
> (Woman, age 84)

The problems patients experienced in recording ECGs underline the vulnerability of those who have simultaneously to cope with a failing body and master a new technology. Patients' experiences also illustrate how they can become careful observers of their own bodies by developing skills to overcome the problems they faced in recording ECGs. This 'artful integration' (Suchman, 2002) included taking the pulse regularly to detect irregularities of the heart rate (Observation telemedical centre, 26 January 2005); forcing an event by walking upstairs three times (man, age 75); doing things that usually trigger heart rate problems (woman, age 72); or recording the ECG on a fixed day of the week after taking a rest (man, age 79). Although patients were thus very creative at handling their problems, not all these approaches can be considered appropriate. Recording only once a week, for example, drastically reduces the chances of capturing irregularities of the heart rhythm. Some patients were even inclined to stop using the recorder because they failed to detect irregularities of their heart rate since these occurred very rarely. They continued to use the device only after the physician who had prescribed the recorder urged them to do so (woman, age 56). Another patient did not use the recorder at all, very much to her regret:

> I did not use it because I often doubted: will I do it or not? Eventually I never did it. Stupid, wasn't it?
>
> (Woman, age 39)

For some patients, acting as a diagnostic agent can thus be so hard that doubt turns into non-use.

The use practices of these patients show another form of articulation work too. Because the work involved in making diagnoses is distributed over several locations, including the home of the patient, patients have to manage another consequence of this distribution: they have to take care of sending the registered ECGs to the telemedical centre. This work turned out to be a challenging task for many patients. Like many other ICTs, the ambulatory ECG recorder combines two technologies: an ECG recorder and a telephone. This convergence of technologies complicates the use of the new device because it requires skills and competencies to master two different machines. Because the telephone is by now a 'relatively naturalised technology' that most people use without paying attention to the intervening medium,[3] we may be inclined to think that it will not impose any barriers to the use of the ECG recorder. The experiences of the patients indicate, however, that an old technology such as the phone has to be mastered anew, when meaning and use become destabilized and modified. Although speaking to someone on the telephone has become part of the routine of our daily life, at least to patients in this research, sending an ECG stored in another machine is a completely novel activity. Sending ECGs via the phone is clearly not considered to be a common, formal property of the telephone. Consequently, this new meaning and use of the technology triggered surprised reactions and distrust among patients, who could not believe that the phone could be used for this purpose. To quote one of the patients:

> After recording you had to dial and you had to put the recorder in front of the mouthpiece of the phone. A bit primitive, I think, but it seems to work.
>
> (Man, age 74)

Other patients only trusted the working of the ambulatory ECG in combination with the phone when they saw the sent ECG in print:

> The first time I thought: this is science fiction! My husband told me that it operates via the satellite. But I thought you are kidding. I did not believe it at all. I only believed it when I visited my general practitioner, who showed me the ECG he had received from the telemedical centre. Then I was convinced that it was real because it was on paper. I simply could not believe that an ECG could be sent via the phone.
>
> (Woman, age 31)

The new use of the telephone also required specific skills: sending the ECG by phone succeeds only if the recorder is put at a certain distance in front of the mouthpiece of the phone. Although this seems to be rather straightforward and simple, this task is more complicated than it seems at first sight because some phones facilitate the sending of ECGs much better than others due to variations in the number and size of the holes in the microphone. Instructions for use could therefore not be standardized and patients had to figure out the optimal distance between the recorder and the phone on their own. The articulation work of patients thus also consisted of learning new skills to coordinate the use of two technological devices and to build trust in the new technology.

Can you hear my heart beat? Patients' invisible work in public spaces

Thus far, my account of patients' invisible work has focused on one specific place: the patient's home. A focus on the home is, however, not enough for understanding how patients try to master the new technology. Although many telecare technologies are designed for home use, some telecare devices, including the ambulatory ECG recorder, are also meant to be used outdoors. Nevertheless, current social science research on the use practices of these technologies only addresses how telecare devices transform patients' homes (Langstrup Nielsen, 2003; Mort et al., 2008; Pols, 2008; Willems, 2010). Consequently, telecare devices meant to be used in public spaces are absent in empirical studies and conceptual discussions of these new technologies. Based on social studies of the mobile phone, we may expect, however, that the use of digital care devices in public spaces seriously affects users as well as spaces. As Cooper (2002) has described, the mobile phone played an important role in blurring the boundaries between discrete domains such as public and private and remote and distant. To capture this blurring of boundaries, he introduced the notion of 'indiscreet technologies' (Cooper, 2002, p. 24). Because mobile phones are by now a widely accepted and domesticated technology in many countries, the ways in which they participate in transforming public spaces are almost taken for granted. In contrast, telecare devices for use outdoors are a more recent development and thus not yet accepted as routine practice, which makes social science research even more interesting and urgent. Equally importantly, the use of digital mobile devices may even be more consequential for its users because it concerns their health rather than communication in general. What happens when patients are expected to use a technology aimed at monitoring and diagnosing their illness in public spaces? What invisible work is involved in using the ambulatory ECG recorder outdoors?

As briefly mentioned above, the ambulatory ECG recorder is meant to be used outside the home. To detect irregularities in heart rhythm, patients are expected always to carry the device with them wherever they go. The articulation work of patients is thus not restricted to their home environment but also involves places such as shopping centres, public transport, or the homes of friends and family. Patients' use practices illustrate the articulation work involved in appropriating mobile telecare devices outdoors. The patients we interviewed all experienced problems in using the ambulatory ECG recorder in public spaces, particularly because of the sound script of this telecare device.

Many new devices, particularly but not exclusively ICT products, are characterized by a lack of transparency in how they work. Designers of telecare devices often anticipate this lack of transparency by designing feedback systems to reassure users that the device is working well. In the case of the ambulatory ECG recorder, patients have to be informed that they have activated the recorder correctly and that the device is storing the ECG for 3½ minutes. Moreover, patients and healthcare professionals at the telemedical centre need feedback from the machine to confirm that the ECGs have been sent and received. Designers chose to base these feedback systems on sound. When the patient pushes the record button, the ECG recorder makes a continuous sound to inform the patient that the recorder is storing the ECG. When the recording is completed, the sound stops. When the patients push the send button, the recorder gives several beeps to signal that the transmission of the ECGs has begun. When the beeps stop, the patient can talk to the physician at the telemedical centre. Beeps are also used to inform the patient about the number of stored ECGs. When the recorder has stored the second ECG, for example; it makes two beeps. When the recorder has stored the maximum number of ECGs (usually four), the recorder gives a continuous beep that lasts a short time to tell the patient that ECGs should be sent to the telemedical centre.[4] The recorder also gives four beeps to inform the user that the batteries are flat or that the memory is full. Failures in the memory of the recorder are also communicated by sound, that is, by repeated beeps when the record button is pushed. Sound signals thus function as an auditory control on various parts of the working of the technology.

Although the script of beeps to invite specific actions or give feedback to users facilitates the use of the ambulatory ECG recorder, the nature of the sound also puts constraints on users. When the recorder stores an ECG, it makes a very sharp, high-pitched, jarring sound. The unintended consequence of this sound script is that it attracts the attention of people close by the user who may wonder what is wrong with that person. Therefore patients are reluctant or may simply refuse to use the recorder outdoors. Many patients experienced the sound as an undesirable transgression of the boundaries between the public and the private. They are afraid that the beeping ambulatory ECG recorder makes their heart problems visible, or in this case audible, to others.[5] Sound signals designed to establish trust thus turn into a violation of patients' privacy: they threaten to disclose health problems to audiences outside the medical domain and the circle of family and friends. In this respect, the ambulatory ECG recorder can thus indeed be considered as an 'indiscreet technology': it has the capacity to transgress boundaries between discrete domains.[6] Patients who do not want these boundaries to be blurred need to do work to bypass the unintended consequences of the sound script of the ECG recorder. The use of the recorder during everyday outdoor activities such as work, travelling in public transport, and visiting family and friends, is therefore considered problematic. To quote some patients:

> I have to go to my work by train and it is, of course, difficult to use [the recorder] there, although it may be necessary to do it. The recorder really raises the roof. It makes an awful lot of noise. Therefore I do not use it when I am not at home.
>
> (Woman, age 56)

> I do not like it that it makes such [a] noise. Sometimes you really think, Should I make an ECG here? You walk in busy streets and you think, Let me wait until I am home again. But then it is actually too late again. During the recording you hear wiew ... wiew ... wiew. You hear your heartbeat, as it were, but pretty hard. Everybody can hear it. Therefore you do not walk at ease there anymore. If it would not make such a noise, I would use it more frequently. I do not want to walk in the supermarket with such a siren.
>
> (Man, age 28)

> When I was in the company of people who were not informed about my complaints and use of the ambulatory ECG recorder, I experienced the sound it made during recording and sending as too loud.
>
> (Woman, age 55)

One patient was so alarmed by the sound of the recorder that she did not trust the technology:

> I thought it was ridiculous. When you make a recording, you hear those tooters and bells. And I was sitting on the settee and I wanted to send it to the doctor, it was the first time, and then it began to beep and rattle. That took five minutes. I really thought, I do not believe at all that you can read my heart rate this way.
>
> (Woman, age 33)

The sound of the ECG recorder is experienced as even more problematic because the recorder can store ECG recordings without the intentional intervention of the user. The record button is so sensitive that it can be activated by the slightest movement of the user, even more so because patients are instructed to wear the recorder at their waistband. Patients could activate the recorder accidentally when they bumped against something or bent or sat down, or because the recorder got jammed at night. Patients became very nervous because they could not stop the recording and had to endure the sound for 2½ minutes before it stopped.[7] Or, as patients put it:

> The buttons are very sensitive. Therefore the recorder can start making a recording by itself. That is a great disadvantage. When I walked in the supermarket, I happened to give it a push and then it began to wail and then you hear your heart beat very loud. Then you do not feel at ease really.
>
> (Man, age 28)

> Once the recorder turned on while I was in the train. I heard a sound and wondered where it came from and discovered it was the recorder. Fortunately it could not make so much noise in my environment because is was hidden under my clothes. But I heard it and I could not switch it off.
>
> (Woman, age 56)

The fact that the ECG recorder could switch on by itself not only made patients nervous because it attracted the attention of others, but also constrained the building of trust in the technology:

> Because of the frequent unintended recordings, I and my family doctor doubted whether the anomalous ECGs could be caused by the apparatus.
>
> (Woman, age 84)

In principle, the problems patients faced with the sound script of the recorder could have been solved by small changes in the artefact. Using light instead of sound as feedback could have been an appropriate solution for patients. However, the producer of the ambulatory recorder does not offer this option (Interview Jurgens, 2004).[8] The responsibility for solving these problems in use were thus delegated to the patients. Patients had to put in quite some effort to 'repair' aspects of the script of the technology that put constraints on its use. To avoid unintended ECGs being made by the recorder itself, some patients were very creative in finding other ways to fix the recorder to their body such as fixing it to the bra, carrying the recorder in a special bag around the back of the neck or in a breast-pocket, clipping it to an elastic waistband, or fixing it at the side of the waistband.[9] However, other patients did not succeed in gaining control over the agency of the ECG recorder, which resulted in a selective use of the technology: they did not wear the recorder during their holiday or took it off during sports, visits, or work, and used the recorder only at home.[10]

The use of sound as feedback to reassure patients of the proper functioning of the recorder also had unintended consequences for a specific group of users. People with hearing deficiencies, predominantly elderly patients, experienced problems in use because they could hardly hear the beeps:

> I have a hearing aid at one side. Sometimes I forgot to wear it and then could not hear the beeps. Therefore they should warn people with a hearing aid that they should activate it. Otherwise you do not hear it when you push the send button. You think: 'does it beep or not?' The beeps are too high for me; that was very difficult. When you are in bed you do not wear the hearing aid. So if you push the button, you do not hear whether you pushed hard enough and whether it worked or not.
>
> (Woman, age 72)

The lack of control among patients with hearing deficiencies often led to failures in recording or sending an ECG. According to the healthcare professionals at the telemedical centre, general practitioners should think twice before prescribing the ambulatory ECG recorder to individuals hard of hearing; otherwise they should take care that there is someone near the patient who can make and send the ECGs (Interview Jurgens, 2004). The choice of the designers to use sound as feedback to users thus has the unintended consequence that people with hearing deficiencies are excluded from use or need assistance from others to become competent users. The sound script of the ECG recorder thus includes an implicit age script: the choice for sound as feedback signal to users assumes users without hearing deficiencies, which are predominantly younger people.

The example of the ambulatory ECG recorder thus shows how design solutions introduced to make up for the lack of transparency of the working of telecare devices can have unintended, negative consequences for users. The use of sound signals to make the working of the telecare device more transparent had serious consequences for people with hearing deficiencies, who became excluded from use or dependent on others. The beeping sounds of this telemonitoring device designed as feedback signals to users also turned the device into a disruptive actor because it made patients' heart problems apparent to others when they used it in public places. The articulation work of patients thus included work to guard the boundaries between the public and the private.

Turning patients into users: The invisible work of home-care nurses

As described above, the use of the ambulatory ECG-recorder requires skills and capacities that are unfamiliar to first-time users. As happened with the metered-dose inhaler for asthma patients described by Prout (1996), the ambulatory ECG recorder-related competencies for patients created new tasks for general practitioners. In the case of the ambulatory ECG-recorder, general practitioners did not do the work required to instruct patients themselves but delegated this task to less-expensive personnel: assistants of the general practitioners and nurses at home-care organizations.[11] The home-care organization is a crucial site for the successful operation of ambulatory ECG recorders: if nurses fail to teach the patients to use the new device correctly, the technology will fail altogether. To be able to perform this task, the nurses themselves have to become acquainted with the new technology. In this sense, home-care-nurses can be seen as the first users of the ambulatory ECG recorder. Like patients' work, the work of home-care nurses consists of visible and invisible work.[12] The visible work of nurses includes the work of instructing patients how to use the ambulatory ECG recorder, a formal task delegated to them during the training they receive from the supplier of the new technology. This instruction work consists of several actions nurses have to perform when patients come to their office to collect the ambulatory ECG recorder. Nurses have to explain how the technology works, including an explanation of the whole procedure from attaching electrodes to the chest, fixing the electrodes to the recorder, and making and sending an ECG. The instructions nurses have to give are not restricted to verbal explanations but also include a demonstration to give patients a first hands-on experience with the new technology.

An exploration of the work of home-care nurses indicates that their role in making this technology work is much broader than that of instructing patients how to use the new technology. Sometimes patients can become very nervous and worried when they realize that they have to operate the ECG recorder themselves. When this happens, nurses have to put quite some effort into comforting and reassuring them that they will be able to master the technology. Other patients object when they hear that they have to carry the device day and night. The nurses have to convince them of the benefits of the new technology by telling the patients how this ECG recorder enables them to produce a continuous registration of their ECG instead of an occasional registration, thus increasing the chances of monitoring irregularities in their heart rhythm (Interview Woudenberg, 2004).

The work nurses do to comfort and reassure patients becomes even more important when they have to instruct patients without much experience with similar digital technologies or patients who have problems with the Dutch language. The nurses' experiences show how the attitudes of patients towards the new technology differ greatly according to age, gender, and ethnicity. Whereas young men considered the ambulatory ECG recorder to be an extremely interesting technology, elderly women, in particular, were very much impressed by what the machine could do but also considered it as a scary apparatus, were afraid to push the buttons, complained about the small size of the batteries, or became nervous when they learned that they had to operate the recorder themselves (Interview Dam en Woudenberg, 2004). Moreover, the Dutch language script of the ambulatory ECG recorder (the instructions, the manual and the phone conversations with the telemedical centre are in Dutch) is sometimes an extra barrier for first-generation immigrants who have not mastered Dutch. Occasionally, these patients take a Dutch-speaking family member with them, usually a daughter. Moreover, nurses sometimes meet resistance among first-generation immigrants because they tend to prefer to receive care instead of doing some of the work themselves (Interview Woudenberg, 2004). Using the ambulatory ECG recorder is much easier for users who have learned the required attitudes and skills in other contexts, and nurses have to do extra work for those patients who do not have previous experience or Dutch language skills. To overcome the language barrier, nurses rely more heavily on showing the ambulatory ECG recorder to the patient and pointing to the illustrations in the manual (Interview Woudenberg, 2004; Interview Tongeren, 2004). Nurses also spend more time in giving instructions to elderly women and men as well as immigrants to make sure that they understand the instructions. They also attune the instructions to the needs of these groups of patients by repeating information or modifying the instructions. Because people in their 70s and 80s have more difficulties remembering the number of recorded ECGs, nurses instruct them to send each ECG separately instead of sending four ECGs together (Interview Dam, 2004).

Reflecting on these work practices of home-care nurses, we can conclude that a substantial portion of their work consists of activities that were not included in the training they received previously. This invisible work consists of comforting and reassuring patients about their abilities to master the new technology. This kind of invisible work can best be described as 'inclusion work' (Rommes, 2002): the work nurses do play a major role in turning patients, including potential non-users, into users.

Setting the patients' minds at ease: The invisible work of telephysicians

Dominant discourses on telecare silence not only the work of patients and home-care nurses, they also neglect the work of telecare professionals. As described in Chapter 3, the ambulatory ECG recorder is embedded in a telemedical centre established by the firm Hartis that introduced the ambulatory ECG recorder onto the Dutch market. The staffing of this telemedical centre consists of 16 part-time healthcare professionals: physicians, industrial medicine practitioners, and basic practitioners who received training in reading ECGs at the centre. During the period of this study, the telemedical centre operated 24 hours per day, seven days a week.[13]

A typical contact between a physician at the telemedical centre and a patient who calls the centre proceeds as follows:

> When the telephysician has answered the phone he[14] asks the caller for the ID number and the number of ECGs he or she will send. When the telephysician has found the file of the caller on his computer he or she asks: X is the name, isn't it? That is a nice name, where does

it come from? While the patient tells his or her story, the physician opens the software program that can register and store ECGs and says: 'I am ready. I count down and then it's your turn. Three, two, one.' The telephysician then watches the screen to see the transmitted ECGs and looks for the paper patient record. On the screen he discovers that a part of the ECG has not been submitted correctly: there are lines that do not show any heart rate. The breakdown takes only a short time and then the other ECGs are transmitted correctly. 'Yes, here we are again,' the telephysician says when he picks up the phone again. He explains to the patient what he has seen on the ECGs: 'The first registration looks pretty calm. I have seen your ECGs before and they usually showed PACs: a premature atrium complex. At the second registration the heart rate was a bit faster but that is all within the normal range. At the third registration I saw a part where your heart began to roll. That could be an auricle fibration. That does not do any harm either. It may be a nasty feeling for you but ... I did not see anything abnormal. The only thing is that you were disconnected for a while. Please mind that the electrodes are properly fixed to the skin and that the plugs are connected. The fourth ECG showed a rhythm that was too fast. What were you doing then? No idea? Well, it is not really harmful.' After ending the phone conversation, the telephysician prints the ECGs and puts them in the paper patient record. He corrects the diagnosis of one of his colleagues because he does not agree with the previous evaluation.

(Observation telemedical centre 26 January 2005)

This phone call vividly illustrates the visible and invisible work of physicians at the telemedical centre. The visible, formal task telephysicians have to do is to receive the ECGs and store them on their computers, to refine the anamnesis they received from the family doctor, to interpret the ECGs, to make a first diagnosis, and fax this to the patients' physician. They also have to file the diagnosis in the paper medical records and also include the printed ECG. A major part of the telephysicians' work is, however, not included in these formal tasks. As we have seen, the task to instruct patients had been formally delegated to home-care nurses. The practices we observed at the telemedical centre indicate, however, that telephysicians also play a role in assisting patients to use the technology correctly. Due to frequent failures in recording and sending of ECGs, telephysicians have become accustomed to give patients clear instructions for use, particularly to patients who call for the first time, patients who have not called for more than a week, and elderly patients (Interview Jurgens, 2005). The countdown before patients are asked to push the send button has become routine practice to make sure that patients have their recorder in the right position on time, which is necessary to receive all submitted information (Observation telemedical centre, 19 January 2005).

The approach telephysicians take is to reassure patients that there is no need to be afraid to use the ECG recorder, thus trying to make patients less nervous (Interview Woudenberg, 2004). The reassuring voice of the physicians often helps patients to build trust in the telecare service:

> Initially I did not trust it. We had never heard about it before. So you do not really trust it. Until you get somebody on the phone. You do not get a choice menu or something but a real cardiologist on the phone. I was really reassured when I got the cardiologist on the line. That there is someone there to control everything at the background. Even if you do not trust the recorder, if you feel pressure on you breast you can call them immediately. And then a cardiologist answers the phone directly, they do not let you wait. He explained what I had to do and then I did it, step by step, and then it worked.
>
> (Woman, age 31)

> When you phone the hospital, you usually get a choice menu; that is really frightening. They also refer you to different departments. Here you could talk to someone directly.
>
> (Man, age 72)

The very fact that there is someone answering the phone, even though it is not a cardiologist but a general practitioner, thus seems to be of crucial importance for patients. For some patients, however, this script provides a constraint because they do not want to bother the telephysicians in vain, which results in selective use: they do not call the centre when they are not sure if their complaint is serious enough or when they experience heart problems at night.[15]

Another part of the invisible work of physicians at the telemedical centre consists of giving patients feedback on their ECGs. Although making a final diagnosis is formally the task and responsibility of the general practitioner who has prescribed the ambulatory ECG recorder, telephysicians are very active in communicating their evaluation of the ECG to patients. Physicians at the telemedical centre use a strategy similar to what they use while encouraging patients to send ECGs: they try to set patients' minds at ease. Reassuring patients by direct feedback on their ECGs is crucial for this category of patient. As McDonalds has described 'the suspicion of heart disease can arouse fear rivalled only by cancer, so that patients can become very alarmed by symptoms thought to be related to the heart' (McDonald et al., 1996, p. 7). Patients who act as diagnostic agents thus experience a double fear: they are nervous because they have to use a new technology and because they are worried about their hearts. The work as physician of a telemedical centre thus requires skills that go beyond registration and analysis: it also requires psychological skills. The telemedical centre we studied has taken this challenge seriously by hiring a psychologist as staff member (Interview Jurgens, 2005). When telephysicians tell patients their evaluation of the ECGs, they always try to be very careful to avoid extra stress. In case of minor heart irregularities, physicians tell the patients that they do not have to worry: 'this is not harmful', you do not need any medical intervention', do not worry, it's nothing serious'. Sometimes, the telephysicians also explain the causes of the irregularities to help patients understand what they feel, for example, that fast heartbeats can be induced by emotions or drugs or minor dysfunctions of the heart (Observations telemedical centre, 19 and 26 January 2005). Some patients thus learned more about their heart problem, which reduced their anxiety. Most patients highly appreciated the direct feedback on their ECGs from the physicians. They praised this personal contact and the fact that they took enough time to discuss the interpretation of the ECGs with them. To quote one patient:

> Each time I called, he [the physician] told me that I did not have to worry. He tried to put my mind at ease and told me that there was no abnormal disturbance. So I accepted this.
>
> (Woman, age 57)

Many patients considered the direct feedback by phone as one of the most important aspects of the technology, even more important than sending the ECGs by phone. Or as one patient put it:

> Of course I want to see or hear results. Sending the ECG is of course a very abstract thing, you see. That does not help me. You want to hear that the ECG is transmitted well and to hear the results. It never

happens that they tell you that they call you back in a half an hour
or so. No, they give you the result at once.

(Man, age 59)

A final important part of the invisible work of physicians at the telemedical centre consists of social work. Many patients make more phone calls
to the telemedical centre than is strictly required to send ECGs. Because
patients have never met the doctor who answers the phone before, the
phone line is used to build relationships with the remote physicians.
During these, sometimes frequent, contacts the patients inform the
telephysicians not only about their heart problems but also about their
other worries. In our interviews, patients told us that they appreciated it
very much that one telephysician in particular devoted so much time to
their stories and that the physician, after several calls, remembered who
they were. Some patients told us that they frequently call not to send
ECGs but for social talk. Occasionally, the phone conversations create
bonds that make patients call back because the telephysician sounded
somewhat depressed during their first call (Observation telemedical
centre, 19 January 2005).

Reflecting on the invisible work of the physicians at the telemedical
centre we can conclude that this work can be considered articulation
work. Telephysicians turn out to be important actors in managing the
consequences of the distributed nature of the work involved in producing diagnoses, consequences that were not foreseen by designers. For
patients this articulation work is of crucial importance to be able to
act as diagnostic agents. The phone contacts with the telephysicians
were important to build trust in the new technology, particulary for
elderly women. The general practitioners could rely on the physicians
at the telemedical centre to provide feedback on the ECG reports and
to discuss whether any intervention was needed. Many general practitioners do not have the required education in cardiology and therefore
put their faith completely in the judgement of the telemedical centre's
physician (Interview Jurgens, 2005). Home-care nurses could rely on
the physicians at the telemedical centre because they could ask them
for help in case they faced practical problems with the ambulatory ECG
recorder that they could not solve themselves (Interview Woudenberg,
2004). The emerging geography of telecare thus depends on different
forms of invisible work for physicians at the telemedical centre. In
addition to articulation work, this new category of healthcare providers
has to perform work that can be described as 'affective work' (Hardt,
1999) to create 'intimacy at a distance'.[16] Although affective work is an

important aspect of healthcare in general, it seems to be more impera-
tive in healthcare at a distance (Wahlberg et al., 2003).

Conclusions

My account of use practices of the ambulatory ECG recorder in the
Netherlands illustrates how telecare technologies redefine the identity
of patients. In the emerging landscape of telecare, patients are configured as diagnostic agents rather than passive recipients of healthcare.
But how can we explain the success of many patients in adopting the
role of diagnostic agent? This question can be answered partly by the
specific situation in which patients are confronted with this new technology. The moment when individuals with heart complaints visit their
general practitioner and receive a prescription for the ambulatory ECG
recorder can be described as a 'fateful moment', a concept introduced
by Giddens to refer to 'moments where consequential decisions are
concerned'. According to Giddens, these periods often mark periods
of reskilling: 'at such moments when life has to be seen anew, it is
not surprising that endeavours at reskilling are likely to be particularly
important and intensively pursued. Where consequential decisions are
concerned, individuals are often stimulated to devote the time and
energy necessary to generate increased mastery of the circumstances
they confront' (Giddens, 1991, p. 96). Individuals visiting their general
practitioner for heart complaints are confronted with decisions that
change the course of their lives. They can become diagnosed as having
serious heart dysfunctions, thus becoming heart patients, or they will
be reassured that everything is normal and they can continue with their
life as usual.

Whereas prior to the introduction of the ambulatory ECG recorder
healthcare professionals performed all the work necessary to make the
decision to categorize individuals as heart patients or not, now patients
are asked to play an active role in this decision. They are expected to
use the ambulatory ECG recorder to provide the general practitioner
with the data to make a diagnosis. This research shows how patients
gradually learned to perceive the ambulatory ECG recorder as a tool
with which to gain mastery of the situation they faced. Like Giddens,
I found that patients were eager to reskill themselves because of the
consequential transitions in their lives. They were motivated to learn
to become competent users and diagnostic agents because this was the
only way in which they could regain mastery of the situation. Another
possible solution could have been to ask for a referral to a cardiologist.

Patients did not choose this alternative because of the long waiting lists for appointments to see cardiologists. Moreover, their general practitioners were eager to try the new technology instead of referring their patients to a cardiologist. The new technology enabled them to keep the patients longer as their own clientele (Interview Hollander, 2004). The use of the ambulatory ECG recorder held the promise that patients would gain insight into the cause of their heart problem and eventually access to a medical treatment. Or, as a patient put it: 'you hold on to every straw' (man, age 59).

However, the question of how patients succeed in adopting the role of diagnostic agent in telecare cannot be understood solely in terms of Giddens' notion of the 'fateful moment'. Giddens conceptualized the ways in which patients learn to use and trust expert systems merely as a psychological, motivational process that operates at the level of interaction of the individual with one specific expert system (Giddens, 1991). Although Giddens discussed the ways in which individuals put faith in expert-based abstract systems, telecare technologies provide a more complex challenge for both patients and sociologists, because they are a conflation of two different expert systems: the medical expert system of healthcare professionals taking care of health complaints, and the technical expert system of ICT innovations in healthcare. Equally importantly, telecare technologies are different from other technologies because they replace face-to-face contacts between healthcare professionals and patients with virtual encounters. Patients are expected to act as diagnostic agents in the absence of healthcare professionals. This is not to say that healthcare professionals don't play any role. Based on a techno-geographical approach, which takes into account the interdependencies among patients, healthcare professionals and technical devices inscribed in telecare technologies, the chapter shows how patients succeed in playing an active role in the diagnosis of their heart problems only because of the support of other actors. First, nurses and general practitioners' assistants facilitate the active role of patients in producing diagnoses because they provide access to the knowledge and skills necessary to use the new technology. Second, the ambulatory ECG recorder helps patients to perform the role of diagnostic agent by giving feedback based on sound signals when patients have completed a task successfully. Last but not least, patients succeed in playing an active role in diagnosis at a distance because of the active support provided by the physicians at the telemedical centre. As we have seen, the telephysicians assisted patients in using the technology correctly, reassured patients about their heart problems, and comforted them when they had other worries. The fact that the ambulatory ECG recorder worked via a phone line to the telemedical centre turned out to be of crucial importance to patients, because it enabled direct contact with these physicians. Digital proximity thus depends not only on novel ICT-based systems. Familiar technologies such as the phone remain important actors in creating intimacy at a distance. We can thus conclude that many patients were able to adopt the role of diagnostic agent not only because of their individual motivation but because of the invisible work of telephysicians and home-care nurses. This work not only consisted of articulation work, but also included affective work and inclusion work.

However, the support of healthcare professionals did not solve all the problems patients encountered in acting as diagnostic agents. My analysis showed important patterns of selective use and non-use that could not be prevented by home-nurses or telephysicians. The sound script of the ambulatory ECG-recorder excluded people with hearing deficiencies, or made them dependent on others, and interfered negatively with using the device outdoors. The fact that the telecare device included use in public spaces required the patients to do extra work: they had to hide its use from others in order to prevent disclosure of patients' heart problems to people outside the close circle of family and friends. Many patients resisted this transgression of boundaries between the public and the private and decided to use the ambulatory ECG recorder only at home. The new technology also redefined patients' relationships to public spaces. The use of the telecare device transformed shopping malls and trains into scary spaces because it could lead to an unwanted exposure of their failing bodies to others.

We can thus conclude that telecare technologies are not per definition inclusive. This chapter has shown how the very design of a technology can transform users into selective users or non-users. The next chapter continues to investigate how telecare technologies may involve non-use by focusing on patients who resisted using telecare devices at home.

8
Inspecting Bodies and Coping with Disease at Home

> Home is not a Machine, Home is for People. Home is
> an emotionally charged and personally furnished cra-
> dle of living – physical space as much as social-cultural
> context and a state of mind.
>
> (Friedewald and Da Costa, 2003, p. 18)

Technologies as new inhabitants of the home

One of the promises of telecare technologies is that healthcare will move partly from the hospital to the home. Telecare technologies are expected to extend the clinical gaze to non-clinical spaces and to non-professionals, that is, patients. These novel technologies thus follow the path of home-care and self-care technologies by taking diagnostic and monitoring procedures outside the hospital and bringing them into patients' homes. As described in the first chapter, there is, however, a major difference between telecare and other home-care technologies. Because telecare technologies are ICT-based, the home becomes electronically connected and integrated within a wider network of health-care, including telemedical centres, hospitals, and general practitioners' rooms.

But what actually happens when homes become electronically wired to healthcare organizations? How does this affect the places we call 'home'? Although we should be careful to avoid a too romantic view of home, human geographers emphasize that the home should not be considered as a tabula rasa, a merely static, physical space. Instead they suggest that homes should be considered as sites of social relations, historically and culturally specific spaces which contribute to shaping people's identities (Angus et al., 2005; Arras et al., 1995; Friedewald and Da Costa, 2003). As human geography, other disciplines have contributed to rethinking the home by countering the view of the home as an objective space that can be understood in terms of standard measurements. Many of these reconceptualizations originate in the field of phenomenology, particularly the work of Maurice Merleau-Ponty (1962), who introduced the notion of home as 'lived space', emphasizing the role of the body as the locus of perception in experiencing the spatial world.[1] Whereas phenomenology emphasizes the perception of spaces, anthropologists draw attention to the actual activities in the home. Mary Douglas, for example, introduced a notion of home in which she characterized it as 'a pattern of regular doings', thus emphasizing the routines and rituals performed in spaces we call home (Douglas, 1991, p. 289). In line with Douglas, Rowles (1993) described the home as 'a preconscious sense of the setting' that people develop over time based on routines performed in the home. Finally, sociologists introduced the notion of home as a 'site of security, familiarity and nurture' (Tuan, 2004). In this approach, the home is viewed as 'haven', a safe place where people can retreat from the outside world and are more or less in control of the actions that take place in that space. Based on these approaches to the home we may expect that telecare technologies will affect the ways in which patients experience their homes. As geographical research of home-based care for frail, older people indicates, the shift towards care at home reconfigures the home by changing the ways in which people identify with the home and shaping the power relations between informal and formal caregivers, including gender relations (Milligan, 2009, p. 23). Feminist scholarship in this field has demonstrated how care has been constructed as a predominantly female activity and responsibility, which may be reinforced by the shift of care to the home because it may contribute to increasing the care work for women. Equally importantly, homes may be experienced differently by women and men (McDowell, 1999; Milligan, 2009). Based on these insights, we may expect that telecare devices cannot simply be inserted into the home without changing the experience and meaning of home, including the gendered social relationships of its inhabitants.

Although human geography and other disciplines thus provide an important perspective on the home, it does not seem to be adequate to conceptualize home in terms of a dualism between home and machine, as the quotation above suggests. Homes are constituted not only by people: quite to the contrary. In our technological culture, homes are increasingly being populated by technical devices. Applying the techno-geographical approach discussed earlier to home and technologies, technical devices can be viewed as new inhabitants of places we call home. We may thus wonder how these newcomers will affect the home. In contrast to other technological inhabitants, such as high-tech home-care technologies (Heaton et al., 2005), telecare technologies may not be highly visible. Whereas high-tech home-care devices often change the use of specific places in the home substantially (an oxygen machine may turn a living room into a bedroom), telecare devices seem, at first glance, less intrusive. Satellites and broadband connections are literally invisible. Electronic blood-pressure meters and scales or ECG-recorder devices can easily be stored in the bedroom. And the TV and phone on which telecare devices often rely are already familiar technologies in the home. This does not imply, however, that these technologies are less important in changing the meaning, practices and experiences of home. People may experience new technologies as unwelcome intruders in the home, even if these devices do not disrupt the physical space of home so drastically. As Maggie Mort and colleagues have suggested for telecare technologies aimed at the surveillance and monitoring of frail elderly people, these devices may have an important impact on how elderly people experience their homes, despite their (compared to assistive technologies such as wheelchairs and lifts) relative physical unobtrusiveness (Mort et al., 2008, p. 67; Milligan et al., 2010, p. 20, 34). This chapter therefore explores what sort of home is constituted and what patient identities are created when the homes of heart-failure patients are electronically connected to healthcare organizations.

The importance of including non-users

To understand how telecare devices transform the home and patient identities, it is important to include non-users of these new technologies in our analysis as well. A focus on non-use enables us to investigate how homes inhabited by telecare devices differ from homes in which patients rely on other monitoring practices, and to consider what kinds of patient identity are created in these two different situations. Equally importantly, a focus on non-users enables us to go beyond a modernist approach to technology as progress in which the adoption and use of new technologies are considered as the norm. Although the previous chapter also addressed non-use, the focus was on a specific type of non-user: that is, people excluded from technology because of its design. This chapter focuses on another category of non-users: people who rejected the use of telecare devices when they were invited to participate in a clinical trial of a telecare device for heart-failure patients in the Netherlands.[2] In contrast to the non-users of the previous chapter, these non-users can be characterized as voluntary. A useful approach to understanding this non-use is to conceptualize it in terms of a self-reflective, significant act. As described in Chapter 2, the dominant discourses on the diffusion of technologies often approach non-use merely in negative terms. People who do not want to use a technology are often described as 'laggards' or 'have-nots' rather than people who make careful, deliberate choices concerning the use of a specific technology (Wyatt et al., 2002; Selwyn, 2003). Conceptualizing non-use as a significant, self-reflective act enables me to avoid an approach that describes non-use merely in terms of a deficit-framework, and to take non-users seriously as relevant actors in shaping the future of technologies.

In addition, I think it is important to emphasize that non-users are not devoid of technologies but choose to rely on other technologies. Non-users of the Internet, for instance, prefer to use other technologies to search for information, as exemplified by the study of Henwood and colleagues on how patients try to find information concerning health issues (Henwood et al., 2003). Non-use should therefore be seen as a relational category: instead of viewing non-use as an irrational, anti-technological or anti-progressive act, I suggest it is important to consider non-use in relation to the use of other technologies people prefer to rely on to perform specific tasks. This approach to non-users enables me to open the black box of technologies whose existence is often taken for granted, sometimes even to such an extent that they are no longer considered as technologies or receive the label of 'mundane technologies'. By taking non-use into account, we can question claims of novelty and try to understand continuities and discontinuities between 'new' and 'old' technologies, thus going beyond the innovative–mundane dichotomy. Therefore I suggest it is important to compare and contrast the experiences and practices of users and non-users of telecare technologies, although my aim is not to define what is novel or innovative[3] but to understand how the participation in different technology-mediated practices constitutes different meanings of home, patient identities, and relations between bodies and technologies.

A focus on non-users of telecare technologies seems to be even more urgent than investigating non-use of consumer technologies, technologies often analysed in user research in cultural and media studies. First, a decision to resist a new technology may be more consequential when it concerns health rather than leisure of other forms of consumption. Second, healthcare technologies involve domestication processes other than consumer technologies. In the case of healthcare technologies, patients do not take the initiative to purchase the technology, a process that, in domestication theory, is considered crucial to the appropriation of technology (Silverstone et al., 1992). Instead, the technology is offered to them by healthcare professionals and, in the case of reimbursement by health-insurance companies (which is often the case in Europe), patients do not have to pay for it and do not become owners of the technology. Given this context, non-use of healthcare technologies should be considered a very explicit and dedicated choice because patients have to decline an offer made by the healthcare professionals they depend on when dealing with important issues concerning health and illness. Whereas non-users of consumer technologies have to resist persuasive commercials, patients have to reject requests from healthcare professionals who will try to convince them that the use of the technology will improve the level of care for their disease.

The shift in care from the hospital to the home inscribed in telecare technologies implies that a rejection of telecare technologies will possibly decrease care for heart-failure patients. Who cares for heart-failure patients who refuse to use telecare technologies? Dominant discourses on telecare technologies make us believe that the decision to use these technologies is a choice for or against monitoring. When I first became interested in telecare technologies, I expected that patients who reject using these devices could not rely on alternative ways of monitoring their health condition when they were discharged from hospital. During one of my first interviews I soon learned that there is a well-established practice of monitoring heart-failure patients supported by specialized nurses. As described in Chapter 6, since the mid-1990s major hospitals in the US, the UK and some European countries, including the Netherlands, have established special outpatient departments known as heart-failure polyclinics, staffed by the newly established nursing specialty of heart-failure nurse. To understand the non-use of telecare technologies, I thus had to follow users of face-to-face monitoring practices at the polyclinic.

In the next section, I describe how the use of heart-failure telemonitoring devices changes patients' homes and identities. The chapter continues to describe how non-users of these telecare devices rejected these transformations, and how their reliance on face-to-face monitoring constituted a different kind of patient and meaning of home. The chapter concludes with a reflection on how telemediated and face-to-face monitoring of heart failure incorporate different geographies of care and technologies of self.

Transforming the home into an electronic outpost clinic

Flashing lights and talking scales: How homes get wired to healthcare organizations

The first change patients experience when they agree to use the heart-failure telemonitoring device is that a technician visits their home to install a broadband connection. This electronic hardware is required to transfer data between patients and the telemedical centre. As described in Chapter 3, patients are expected to measure their weight and blood pressure daily by using a wireless automated scale and blood-pressure meter. The broadband connection, together with a so-called set-top box, supports the transmission of these measurement data between patients' homes and the telemedical centre, the connection between patients' TV and the Internet, and the communication between patients and healthcare providers at the telemedical centre. The patient's home thus becomes inhabited by various electronic devices, which have to find a place in the household. The set-top box is usually installed near the TV in the living room, whereas the electronic scale and the blood-pressure meter are put in the bedroom (Observations in patients' homes, 2006).

So how do these inhabitants 'behave' in their new environments? The set-top box is a very active presence in the room. When the telemedical centre sends a message to patients' homes, the box gives an orange light signal to notify users that the telemedical centre has received their measurement data, which can be watched on the video channel of their TV set in the form of graphs, representing their measurements over a period of 30 days. The set-top box also gives a flashing light signal to tell patients that they have to watch educational videos on diet or exercise for heart failure, or to fill in a questionnaire as soon as these are sent to their TV. If they do not read the message within a day (telenurses can see in the system whether patients have opened the message), they receive a phone call from the telemedical centre and the light signal will keep flashing; also, when patients watch only part of a video. Although less visible than the set-top box, the TV also provides a new element in the living room. Whereas the TV set was introduced in the home as a technology for entertainment or information, the wireless connection of patients' homes to a telemedical centre transforms the familiar technology into a health device. Instead of watching the news, movies, or other entertainment programmes, patients can watch graphs representing diagnostic markers of their health condition, look at educational videos on their illness, or read messages from telenurses. Finally, the electronic scale introduced in the bedroom also draws attention. Compared to other scales, it is bigger in size because the scale is put into a metal frame, which helps patients to stand still while using the scale. Moreover, the electronic scale can talk! As we will see below, this intriguing feature invites unintended interactions with family members visiting patients' homes.

The active presence of the set-top box and the electronic scale, as well as the changed identity of the TV, helped patients to domesticate the new 'inhabitants' of their home. As Silverstone and colleagues have described, showing a new technology to your family or friends, a process called conversion, is an important aspect of 'taming' technologies (Silverstone et al., 1992). Two features of the telemonitoring system turned out to be very helpful in this process. First, the fact that graphs of patients' measurements of weight and blood pressure could be watched on TV enabled patients to show this to family members or friends who came to visit them. Because the TV and the set-top box were situated in the living room, patients often showed it to their visitors, or sometimes visitors were curious about what the 'small box near the TV' (the set-top box) was doing there and wanted to see the graphs.[4] Although many visitors were often impressed by the new technology, particularly by the fact that it was wireless and that measurements sent from patients' home were transferred to another city (Zwolle: the location of the telemedical centre) and then appeared on the TV set, others were rather critical. For example, the son-in-law of one of the patients, who happened to be a physician, considered the system as too much of a burden for patients (Interview male patient, aged 74).

Another feature of the telemonitoring system that attracted the attention of visitors, particularly children, was the electronic scale. The scale not only showed the measured weight on a display but also used a voice, which said: 'Mister X [name of the patient], you should stand still for a moment.' After a while the voice continued with 'You can step off the scale now', and 'Your weight will be shown in kilograms'. The grandchildren of one of the patients were so fascinated by the talking scale that they wanted to use it each time they stayed with their grandparents, which their grandfather tried to avoid because the data were automatically sent to the telemedical centre (Interview male patient, age 70). The introduction of telecare devices in the home thus changed the experience of home, for both visitors and family. The new devices created an environment in which watching health messages on TV, playing with electronic scales, and discussing the (dis)advantages of telecare devices became part of the visits of family and friends.

Consequently, the heart problems of the user of the telecare device gained a more active presence in patients' homes.

Reorganizing home-time and disciplining bodies

The introduction of telecare devices in the home not only shapes the visitors' and family's experience of patients' homes; it first and foremost changes the experience of patients themselves. As soon as the telecare system is installed in their house, patients are expected to integrate its use into their daily routines. Patients soon learn that being at home is no longer as it used to be prior to the entrance of new technical inhabitants. The new technology is not just another object in the home: the telecare device introduces a techno-geographical configuration of care in which the home is transformed into a place where patients are made responsible for monitoring their bodies. Consequently, patients have to become disciplined to monitor their own bodies. A first step in this process of disciplining patients is that they are expected to observe very precise schedules. Each morning they have to measure their weight on the electronic scale and take their blood pressure. Patients showed us how they had integrated the use of the devices into their daily routines. In order not to forget to take the measurements, most patients had installed the electronic scale and blood pressure meter in their bedroom, so they were reminded to measure their weight and blood pressure when they woke up in the morning. Because they were instructed to take measurements when their bodies were still relaxed and not stressed yet by too much physical movement, they developed the routine of measuring their weight and blood pressure before or shortly after breakfast. Consequently, the morning is broken down into rather fixed time sequences: wake-up, get out of bed, wash yourself, measure your weight and blood pressure, have breakfast. Although the order of the last three activities may vary per patient, the use of the heart-failure system introduces a new element into mornings spent at home.

The telemonitoring device structures not only the early parts of the day. The flashing light of the set-top box and the phone calls of the telemedical centre require the full attention of the patient the whole day through. Patients are expected to switch on their TV as soon as the set-top box gives an orange signal that invites them to look at specific messages. Moreover, patients also have to answer phone calls from telenurses. As described in Chapter 3, the telemonitoring system will send patients and telenurses a message when the system detects deviant measurements. Consequently, nurses will phone patients to ask them why they deviated from the set standards for weight or blood pressure and, if necessary, will ask the clinic to change medication. The telecare device thus not only restructures the patients' time in the morning; it intervenes in their activities during the whole day. This is in sharp contrast to the promises articulated by the producer, Philips, which has suggested that 'patients only have to spend a few minutes each day at their convenience interacting with Motiva [the name of this telecare device, N.O.] (Philips Press Information, May 8 2006). The use of the telecare device definitely takes more than just a few minutes of a patient's time, and patients are not free to choose when to do their measurements or to interact with the telemedical centre. Consequently, the use of the telecare device requires that patients remain at home all day. The script of the technology thus assumes that patients are home bound, which may be the case for often elderly patients who suffer from a severe form of heart failure but not necessarily for patients with a milder form of the disease.

The technology thus requires an immediate form of presence, which can best be described as an asymmetrical tele-co-presence. Following Goffman's notion of co-presence, which referred to physical nearness in social interactions, Zhao has described social interactions mediated by ICTs as tele-co-presence (Goffman, 1959; Zhao, 2005). In many ICT applications, such as the mobile phone and Internet, this digital co-presence is symmetrical. In the case of telecare technologies, however, it concerns an asymmetrical tele-co-presence: patients are always accessible, available, and subject to the physician or the nurse. In contrast, healthcare professionals are not directly accessible and available to patients. Although patients sometimes call the telemedical centre, they are not encouraged to do this. The script of the technology implies that telenurses will call patients in the case of deviant measurements and not vice versa.[5] This asymmetry also includes weekends. Whereas patients are expected to send their data seven days a week, the telemedical centre operates only on weekdays (Interview Borst, 2006). A patient told us that he had received a phone call from the telenurses on a Monday when he had forgotten to send his data that Sunday (Interview male patient, age 74). Some users were very disappointed by this restricted surveillance because they often had heart-failure problems during the weekend, since it was harder for them to adhere to the diet regime at dinners they enjoyed with family or friends (Interview male patient 1, age 70). In the case of problems during weekends patients have to rely on their family doctors (who often do not want to interfere in the care trajectory) or, in case of urgency, visit the hospital (Interviews male patient 1, age 70 and male patient 2, age 70).

Summarizing, we can conclude that the use of the heart-failure monitoring system requires the immediate presence and agency of patients. Patients are expected to use telecare devices at specific moments of the day and to be available for feedback by telenurses all day. The script of this telecare device thus turns its use into a compulsory rather than a voluntary act. As already described in Chapter 6, the telecare device for heart-failure patients transforms self-care into an obligation. The new technology forces patients to comply with the guidelines for medication, diet, and exercises, otherwise nurses will correct them immediately based on the 'flags' nurses receive on their computer screens when patients exceed the set standards for weight and blood pressure. The introduction of telecare technologies into the home thus transforms patients into 'assistant medical personnel', who actively participate in monitoring their own bodies (Langstrup Nielsen, 2003, p. 16).

Redefining gender relations and illness

The techno-geographical configuration in which the monitoring of bodies is delegated to patients at home affects not only patients. The daily inspection of bodies also includes the active involvement of other inhabitants of the home, usually the patients' partners. We became aware of this during our interviews and observations at patients' homes. Initially, our main interest concerned the patient, but soon we learned that husbands or wives played an active role in using the devices as well. It frequently happened that the partner, who was often present during our visit, joined in the conversation and told us very interesting things we would not have noticed had we focused exclusively on the person expected to use the device. This telecare device thus does not only affect individual patients, it also redefines social relations in the home. As Pascale Lehoux et al. (2004) have described for high-tech home-care technologies, other members of the household are often also affected by the introduction of healthcare technology in the home. Technologies used at home may afford or deny specific social relations, and, as I will show, gender relations in particular. During the interviews we learned that the telecare device enabled male partners to act as the 'owner' of the telecare devices ('I had some flashing lights under the TV') and showing their technical competence by answering questions about how the system operated before their wives, the intended users of this telecare device, could tell their story.

However, the most important way in which the telecare device transforms gender relationships in the home is that patients' partners are turned into co-inspectors of bodies. As described above, the telecare device disciplines patients to take care of their bodies at a specific time of the day, a process in which patients' partners play an important role. They often ask whether their wife or husband has conducted the measurements, how high or low their measurements are, or they alert them when they discover the flashing light on the set-top box. Equally importantly, most patients watch the graphs on TV showing their weight and blood pressure measurements, often together with their partner. This joint watching enabled them to share with their partner how successful they were in adhering to the set standards, which are displayed on the screen by a firm line representing the upper and lower limits of weight and blood pressure. Again, there are specific gender dynamics at work. The male partners of female patients seem to be particularly keen to assist their wives to operate the telecare system, as is exemplified by the experiences of a female patient:

> Of course I have my husband, but with the system you know that you are not standing alone. That was reassuring. When there was a message and the lights flashed, my husband always checked immediately whether it was important.
>
> (Interview female patient, age 69)

The support of her husband in using the telecare system made her more confident to cope with her disease at home. Like this patient, another female patient also felt reassured by the presence of the telecare device because it reduced her worries. Although initially she did not like the system because she received too many phone calls from the telenurses, she began to appreciate the new presence in her home:

> It feels like you have a doctor at home each day. There is, as it were, a doctor around you. I thought it important that there was someone watching me all the time.
>
> (Interview female patient, age 71)

Although the doctor was never physically there, and the system worked with nurses, for this patient the technology meant the omnipresence of a doctor. Consequently, she worried less about her condition and did not visit her family doctor so frequently as she used to do before she used the telemonitoring devices (Interview female patient, age 71).

Whereas male patients supported their wives in interacting with the telecare device, the role of female partners is more directed towards taking care of bodies rather than technical devices. Female partners supported their husbands in adhering to dietary instructions aimed at avoiding too salty food, which is bad for their health condition. Male patients told us stories about how their spouses used the recipes provided by video messages of the telecare system to prepare healthy meals. Most importantly, female partners also assisted their husbands to cope with their emotions. Male patients often shared their anxiety over the results of the measurements with their partners, as is exemplified by this male patient:

> I often look at the blood pressure and then I think: 'damn, it is not as it should be for a week already.' Then I am rather far above the line, whereas I should be far below it ... Then I tell my wife about it and I wonder what will happen to me again that day. If I had not seen it, I would not have known it.
>
> (Interview male patient 1, age 70)

As Henwood and Wyatt have described for patients searching for health information on the Internet, for patients 'ignorance is bliss sometimes' (Henwood et al., 2003). For this patient, close scrutiny of his body reinforced his experiences of a failing body. He considered it as a burden to watch the messages and graphs all the time, particularly at times when he did not feel very well, and relied on his wife to cope with confronting messages. This supporting role put quite some pressure on female partners. For some of them, the information provided by the TV increased their anxiety, as is illustrated by this female partner:

> Sometimes I consider it as too much of a burden because I worry when the measurements are too high. I begin to look for a reason immediately. I want to know who is to blame. Sometimes I think that we have been too busy. Or: 'you should not eat too much'. Then I try to find a cause, but there is not always a reason, of course.
>
> (Interview female partner of male patient, age 74)

The patient's wife thus considered it as her responsibility when her husband failed to meet to the standards set for weight, which made her feel guilty. The disciplining script of the technology is thus not restricted to the patient but can also affect partners in a very specific gendered way. For this female partner the technology introduced a guilty self.

The use practices of the heart-failure telemonitoring system in patients' homes thus illustrate how this telecare device supports specific gender dynamics in this techno-geographical configuration of care.

Although the telecare system turned male as well as female partners into co-inspectors of their spouses' bodies, the way in which they adopted this role was remarkably different. Whereas male partners supported their wives to interact with the telecare system, female partners assisted their husbands in adhering to their dietary instructions and in coping with emotions related to the results of monitoring their illness.

The active involvement of patients and their partners in monitoring heart failure affects not only their relationship but also how they cope with illness and failing bodies at home. By using telecare devices, patients' bodies become a source of objectified medical knowledge, not only for healthcare professionals bout also for patients and their partners. Knowing their bodies and coping with illness at home are no longer restricted to patients' subjective experience of health and illness, but are also shaped by measuring weight and blood pressure. Patients' measurements, the graphs, and the phone calls collectively produce a body that is known and controlled in terms of weight and blood pressure. The telemonitoring system thus changes what it means to be a heart-failure patient. As a heart-failure patient, you will have to pay attention to your weight and blood pressure daily by taking measurements and keep these bodily indicators within the set limits by taking your medicines and adhering to a bodily regime of diet and exercises. Heart failure is thus no longer only experienced and practised as a disease of the heart but becomes a condition that interferes with, and can be controlled by, taking care of your weight and blood pressure. To take care of your heart, you should take care of your weight and blood pressure. As Willems has described for chronic lung diseases, monitoring practices can thus be considered as practices in which diseases acquire new characteristics (Willems, 1998, p. 115). This does not mean that these characteristics emerge only by using the telemonitoring system. As I will describe below, taking care of your weight is also an important aspect of face-to-face monitoring programmes. Nevertheless, the awareness of heart failure as a disease that can be controlled by taking care of your weight and blood pressure becomes more powerful when it is embedded in a telecare system that disciplines patients to control their weight and blood pressure daily than when it only figures in information leaflets or educational videos. Heart failure as a disease that can be controlled by weight and blood pressure measurements becomes more real and persuasive by using a telemonitoring system, particularly one based on compulsory compliance.

These use practices of the heart-failure telemonitoring system in patients' homes thus illustrate how this telecare device introduces a specific configuration of social relations that is not only characterized by a specific gendered division of labour but also by an uneven distribution of responsibilities and control. In contrast to the promises articulated by the producer of this telecare device, which suggests that the technology enables patients to 'manage their disease themselves', the technology participates in introducing a practice of self-care in which technical devices, telenurses, patients, and their partners collectively 'manage' heart-failure disorders.

Although all the actors play a role in monitoring the condition of heart-failure patients, the control over this process is delegated to telecare devices and telenurses. The conversion of homes into electronic outpost clinics thus transforms patients into subjects that are acted upon: patients are constituted as dependent on the technology and on healthcare professionals.

Monitoring heart failure at the policlinic and at home

Diaries, physical observations, and the self-disciplined patient

As described in the introduction to this chapter, not all patients embrace the introduction of telecare devices in their homes. Some patients who were invited to participate in the clinical trial organized to introduce the telecare device in Europe refused to use the new technology. Instead, they preferred the alternative way of monitoring their body provided by the heart-failure polyclinic.

The face-to-face monitoring programme of these clinics represents a very different geography of responsibilities from the telemonitoring practice described above. In the face-to-face monitoring programme, inspection of bodies is a shared responsibility of patients and heart-failure nurses. Instead of delegating responsibility and control to telecare devices, patients use other, more low-tech technologies. Patients are expected to keep a diary of their weight (blood pressure is not included in this form of monitoring). This technology enables patients to monitor whether their weight remains more or less stable for a week, or whether there are outliers. In addition to diaries of weight, some patients keep records of what they eat to control their intake of salt (Interview female patient, age 66). Although patients thus have to monitor their bodies in the absence of the healthcare professionals, heart-failure nurses instruct patients to call them if they notice a sudden increase in weight or other symptoms that indicate a worsening of their heart-failure, such as swollen legs, shortness of breath, or pain in the chest, which patients often do (Interview heart-failure nurse B; interview Balk, 2007). Patients are also expected to visit the heart-failure nurses at the policlinic every 2–3 weeks, or once every six weeks, depending on the phase of their illness. During these visits, nurses will observe the physical condition of patients, control patients' diaries on their weight, refer patients to diet specialists in the hospital, give emotional support, or refer patients to special meetings for psychological help, or ask for laboratory tests.

The regular visits to the heart-failure polyclinic were one of the reasons why patients rejected the use of telecare devices. Patients told us that they preferred the physical co-presence of the heart-failure nurses. They did not want to lose the visits to the polyclinic because they appreciated the personal contact with the heart-failure nurses, their availability (a visit can be arranged often the same day), and because the personal contact made them feel more secure and less anxious, particularly because of the positive feedback and advice they received. As one male patient told us:

> The personal contact with the heart-failure nurse is very important. I would not like to miss an appointment, because this is really very important for me. I prefer to talk to her personally rather than through the phone. Personal contact works much better. My heart-failure nurse knows me very well. She can tell by looking at my face how I am doing that day, whether I am doing fine or not.
>
> (Interview male patient, 57)

Personal contact is thus very important for this patient, as well for a female patient who told us that she had established a very friendly, trusting relationship with her heart-failure nurse:

> I have a real[ly] trusting relationship with her on a very friendly basis. She will come up with things and then I will mention something. I really like this face-to-face contact; phones and telemonitoring devices are so [im]personal. You cannot express your feelings. But I can express them at the heart-failure nurse. I am not such an advocate of these technologies. For me it is the personal contact that matters
>
> (Interview female patient, age 66)

The major reason for patients' refusal to use telecare devices was, however, that they wanted to keep the responsibility for inspecting their bodies as much as possible in their own hands. They fiercely resisted the dependency and compelled compliance scripted in the telecare system. As one female patient told us:

> I do not want to use the telemonitoring system because you are obliged to use it always at the same moment. You lose a part of your freedom. And I do not want to be controlled always and everywhere. I think it comes down to Big Brother is Watching You. I am still young and independent and do not want to be controlled everywhere. I want to keep my life in my own hands as long as possible.
>
> (Interview female patient, age 48)

Another female patient expressed similar concerns:

> I do not need any devices by which they can control my weight. I watch it myself. When it is too extreme I will ask for help. When there is an extreme change within one day, I retain fluid. I do not have to measure myself daily at the same time on a scale. Sometimes I measure myself when I wake up, but not every day, only to know how I am doing. When I want to know something specific, I will look for it on the Internet.
>
> (Interview female patient, age 66)

A male patient also relied primarily on himself supported by his scales, not only to monitor his weight but also to adhere to the bodily regime of diet:

> I follow my own judgements and also my scale. I will skip it sometimes but usually I will measure my weight each morning. A difference in weight implies fluid. When I gain two kilograms, it is simply two kilograms of fluid. I know that I have to adhere to my diet, that I cannot eat three of four salt herrings because then I will retain fluid. I notice this immediately.
>
> (Interview male patient, age 57)

The experiences of these patients exemplify how patients reject the sort of life implicated in using telecare devices at home. These devices are not simply considered as another handy tool in the household, which requires only a few minutes of attention every day; they are perceived as tools that make patients dependent on healthcare professionals. Some patients also rejected the use of the telemonitoring system because the daily surveillance created a constant awareness of their disease, which threatened their sense of self. Patients told us that they did not want to be confronted with their illness all the time. Or, to quote a female patient:

> You do not want to be reminded about it [heart failure, N.O.] continuously, because you have to pick up your life again. Of course, it is there, but you do not have to bother 24 hours a day. You have to try to return to your normal life rhythm.
>
> (Interview female patient, age 48)

Another female patient expressed similar concerns:

> I do not want to use any medical equipment such as a blood pressure meter because I am afraid that I will begin to measure my blood pressure each morning. Then I do not live so pleasantly anymore, so I resist it. You will begin to compare everything and feel everything. I do not want this to happen, I do not want to become anxious. I do not feel anything right now and I do not want to bother about it, with all my heart.
>
> (Interview female patient, age 66)

These patients thus refuse to become a permanently ill body or, to quote this patient again:

> Last Monday my grandchild asked me whether I was still ill. I told her that I am not ill but that my heart does not function so well anymore. And that I could not jump so well anymore, etc. Th[ose] sort of things I cannot do anymore. But I do not feel myself a heart patient, I do not feel that way.
>
> (Interview female patient, age 66)

Non-users of the telemonitoring system thus resist the daily surveillance of the telecare technology because it creates an omnipresence of their disease, which results in a distorted image of self. They resist a conflation between the self and their failing body.

The monitoring practices at the polyclinic and patients' homes thus constitute patients as self-disciplined individuals who want to remain in control of their own bodies. Although inspecting bodies is a collective responsibility of patients and heart-failure nurses, patients have to rely on their own discipline, experience, and judgement to control their weight and to adjust their lives to the bodily regime of medication, diet, and exercise. The polyclinic does not provide patients with specific guidelines or precise schedules for monitoring their condition. Patients who are in a more or less stable condition are advised to measure their weight twice a week, whereas patients who are less stable are asked to take more frequent measurements (Interview heart-failure nurse A, 2006). Patients are responsible not only for measuring and registering their weight; they also have to interpret these measurements themselves. The monitoring practices at the polyclinic thus reveal a different geography of responsibilities from the telemonitoring practices described above. Whereas the telemonitoring system delegates the interpretation of weight and blood pressure to the technical system and telenurses, patients who rely on face-to-face monitoring have to decide all by themselves what a certain measurement means, what they should do to reduce their weight, or whether they should contact the policlinic to ask for help (Interviews heart-failure nurses A and B, 2006).

Protecting boundaries between the home and the clinic

The rejection of telecare devices by heart-failure patients cannot be understood only in terms of a resistance to becoming dependent on healthcare professionals. Non-users also resisted the transformation of their homes into an electronic outpost of the clinic. To them, home is a place where you want to be free to do whatever you like. In this respect, the stories patients told us confirm Mary Douglas's view of the home as a place characterized by routines. Patients considered the telecare device as an unwelcome inhabitant of the home because it disrupts their daily life pattern and routines at home. As one male patient told us:

> I consider it as an extra burden and I do not like that because I want to be free. When I want to look for something in my study, then it is a beautiful chaos, then I do not want to measure my blood pressure in the meantime. It (taking measurements, N.O.] interferes with what you planned to do. In the morning I want to read my newspaper, then I do not want to think: 'I should do it again.' And then you have all those phone calls. It only gives you extra work. I lived for 86 wonderful years, so let me live and enjoy what there is with a little bit more effort.
>
> (Interview male patient, age 86)

Patients not only value and defend their freedom at home, they also do not want any restrictions in their mobility. As described above, the telecare technology can be used only at home and thus assumes that patients are always at home. If patients do not measure and send their weight and blood pressure data daily, telenurses will phone them immediately. Some patients resist becoming home bound. They want to spend the weekends at the campsite, stay over for a night when they visit their grandchildren or friends, or have a short holiday with their children when they feel well (Interviews male patients 57 and 87; interview heart-failure nurse A, 2006).

But there is more at stake than a resistance to the technology's intrusion into the daily lives of patients. Patients also refused to use the telecare devices because they wanted peace of mind while being at home. In this respect, patients' experiences are in line with the view of home as 'haven', a safe place where people can retreat from the pressures of the outside world and are more or less in control over what happens there. Telecare technologies seem to threaten this secure place. As one female patient told us:

> I do not want to have all that equipment in my house. That is all too much for me. I want peace of mind. That's why I said no. They wanted to give me a scale and a blood pressure meter, but I told them that I do not suffer from tightness anymore, but that I want peace. I do not want to commit myself to anything at this moment.
>
> (Interview female patient, age 66)

For this patient, home is a place of contemplation, a sanctuary that is threatened by telecare devices. The experience of this female patient, and some of the patients cited above, illustrates how patients actively defend the boundaries between home and the clinic. To them, home is a place where you do not want to be a heart patient all the time. These patients experienced telecare devices first and foremost as devices that bring the clinic into their home, a transformation they rejected because it threatened their independence and freedom.

Conclusions

My account of telemonitoring and face-to-face practices of heart failure shows how introducing telecare devices into the home has far-reaching consequences. The introduction of this new technology involves much more that just using a medical device for a couple of minutes a day, as the producer of this telecare device for heart-failure patients promised potential users. The use of the heart-failure telemonitoring system implied that patients' homes became electronically connected to a telemedical centre, thus transgressing the boundaries between the home and the clinic. This 'home–hospital hybrid', to use Dick Willems's felicitous phrase, included a redefinition of the home and relationships within the home (Willems, 2008). Patients' homes became adjusted to the aesthetics and routines of the clinic and patients' partners were turned into co-inspectors of patients' bodies. In this respect, there are important gender dynamics at play. On the one hand, telecare devices act as 'gender benders' because they participate in delegating responsibilities for taking care of health problems to both women and men. In this way, the technical device disrupts traditional gender relations in which women bear the major responsibility for healthcare work in the home, ensuring their husbands and children take medication or adhere to special diets or a healthy lifestyle (Annandale and Kuhlmann, 2010). The introduction of the telecare system in the home can be considered a drastic intervention in this gendered division of healthcare work because the task of monitoring their health condition is delegated to men as well as women.

Nevertheless, some of the traditional gender relations remain firmly in place. Although the telecare devices transform both women and men into co-inspectors of their partners' bodies, men and women adhere to a traditional division of care work in which male partners assist their wives in using the technical device and women support their husbands in coping with emotions and adhering to diets.[6]

The introduction of the heart-failure telemonitoring system not only transformed the home and the role of patients' partners; it also introduced a geography of responsibilities that redefined patient identities and the relationship between technologies and bodies. To understand the different ways in which telecare and face-to-face care affect patients' bodies and identities, it is useful to adopt Foucault's notion of the technologies of self. Foucault has introduced this term to refer to processes in which different forms of self emerge in different practices: 'as there are different forms of care, there are different forms of self' (Foucault, 1998, p. 22). Although Foucault restricted himself to studying technologies of self as performed in ancient Greek and early Christian culture, in which he showed how 'taking care of yourself', in addition to 'knowing yourself' were important aspects of these cultures (Foucault, 1988, p. 19), his concept of the technologies of self is also very useful for analysing monitoring practices in twenty-first century healthcare. There is, however, as Dick Willems has suggested already, an important difference between current monitoring practices and the technologies of self studied by Foucault – namely, their reliance on technical devices (Willems, 1995, p. 122) The self that emerges in monitoring practices in modern healthcare is not constituted by introspection of the soul, like the technologies of self described by Foucault, but is created in networks of care in which patients, healthcare professionals, and technical devices are collectively involved in measuring, controlling, and intervening in bodily functions. Monitoring practices thus function as the technologies of self that rely on measurements of the body rather than introspection of the soul. Despite this difference between Foucault's objects of study and current monitoring practices in healthcare, there is an important similarity as well. According to Foucault, the technologies of self are explicitly medical: 'the care of the self isn't another kind of pedagogy; it has to become permanent medical care'. Permanent medical care is one of the central features of the care of the self. 'One must become the doctor of oneself' (Foucault, 1988, p. 31). In monitoring practices for heart-failure patients there is a similar concern for permanent medical care in which patients are expected to participate in the practice of self-monitoring to enable daily surveillance (in the case of telemonitoring) or intermittent surveillance (in the case of face-to-face monitoring) of bodily functions. As Willems has described for self-monitoring programmes for chronic asthma patients, monitoring practices that delegate part of the responsibility for surveillance of the body to patients involve not only the delegation of tasks from the doctor to the patient; they also constitute the emergence of new patient identities, or forms of self (Willems, 1995, p. 122).

Although both the monitoring technologies investigated in this chapter help patients to take care of themselves, they constitute very different relationships between bodies, technologies, and self. The bodies of patients who use the telemonitoring system become objects for technological devices, experts, and themselves: bodies that are always available and accessible, not just to their own family doctors or cardiologists and their partners, but also to a network of healthcare professionals they will never meet in person. Although patients become actively involved in gazing into their own bodies, my analysis shows how heart-failure telemonitoring devices delegate a rather restricted form of control to patients. The telecare device forces patients to comply with the guidelines for medication, diet, and exercise, otherwise nurses will correct them immediately. Although patients do the measurements themselves, the telemonitoring system 'stands in' for control over their weight and blood pressure, taking away part of the patients' responsibility. Patients remain responsible for measuring weight and blood pressure and adhering to the medical regime, but the control and interpretation of their bodily data is delegated to the system and healthcare professionals. The telecare system thus constitutes the patient as dependent. Moreover, the heart-failure monitoring system can be considered as a specific form of the technologies of self in which taking care of your weight and blood pressure becomes the central element. Equally important, this form of care makes the body into a permanently ill body that needs to be controlled by daily surveillance.

The bodies of patients who participated in the face-to-face monitoring programme remain objects for themselves, assisted by, but not dependent on, medical experts or technical devices. Patients are not only responsible for measuring their weight; they also have to interpret these measurements themselves and take the initiative to ask for medical assistance if their condition becomes worse. The face-to-face monitoring programme thus constitutes the patient as independent: patients remain responsible for their own well-being. This was also the reason why patients participating in the face-to-face programme rejected the use of the heart-failure monitoring system: they resisted the compulsory compliance and dependency scripted in this technology and wanted to keep responsibility for monitoring their condition in their own hands. In contrast to the telemonitoring system, the monitoring of patients' condition was not restricted to bodily indicators such as weight and blood pressure but also included other characteristics of the disease, including psychological aspects. This form of taking care of yourself thus resembles Foucault's technologies of self, which include the introspection of the soul (Foucault, 1988). Finally, the relationship between body and self that emerges in the face-to-face monitoring shows a clear separation between the self and the failing body: the technology helps patients to resist a conflation between the self and their illness.

We thus can conclude that telemonitoring devices and face-to-face monitoring for heart-failure patients incorporate different geographies of care, which support different technologies of self. Whereas the use of telecare devices constitutes patients as dependent on healthcare professionals and redefines the home as an extension of the clinic, face-to-face monitoring reflects a practice of inspecting bodies in which patients are constituted as independent and the home as a distinct space that should not become intertwined with the clinic.

Conclusions: The Importance of Place, Proximity and Diversity

Technological devices can do and mean a lot. My argument throughout this book has been that telecare technologies cannot be considered as isolated instruments that can simply be implemented and diffused in healthcare without changing the order of care and what care is all about. The previous chapters have illustrated how telecare technologies participate in actively transforming healthcare by creating different forms of care, redefining professional and patient identities, and introducing a new category of healthcare professionals and a new healthcare organization. Reflecting on the techno-geographical approach introduced in this book, I conclude that this approach has provided an appropriate heuristic for understanding how technology-mediated connections between places, actors, and technical devices change the landscape of healthcare. It is time to summarize and reflect on the major findings of this study.

De-centring the clinic? Distributing and controlling the clinical gaze

Technologies do not work by themselves. In contrast to what advocates of telecare technlogies promise, these new devices do not reduce human labour. As I have described in this book, the introduction of this new technology involves a proliferation in the care work required to produce, read, and interpret diagnostic and monitoring data, to instruct patients on how to use telecare devices, and to integrate the new technology into patients' homes and telemedical centres. The implementation and use of telecare technologies for heart patients implies that more actors are becoming involved in healthcare, including cardiologists, heart-failure nurses, general practitioners, home-care nurses, telenurses, telephysicians, health insurance companies, telemedical firms, and, last but not least, patients. Although the future of the new technology thus depends on many different people who are expected to do often novel work, some actors and work remain largely invisible in the dominant discourses on the new technology. In this book I have attempted to make up for these absences by focusing on the work of two of these silenced actors: telecare workers and patients. The techno-geographical approach developed in this book has enabled me to draw attention to the ways in which technological devices delegate tasks and responsibilities to people and devices, thus producing specific geographies of responsibility (Akrich, 1992). As suggested in Chapter 2, a conceptualization of these changes in terms of geography rather than network is important to highlighting the fact that the distribution of responsibilities and work among users of technologies takes place between actors that are not equally situated or represented in discourses on healthcare. Whereas the metaphor of a network assumes non-hierarchical relations among humans and between technological objects and people, the term 'geography' makes us sensitive to distributions of responsibilities and work which grant agency and power to specific actors while restricting or silencing the agency of others.

Let me first summarize my major findings on the work of telecare professionals. Telecare workers can be considered as an intriguing category of healthcare professionals: they do not have their own discipline or work domain but act as intermediaries in healthcare. As we have seen, their work consists of mediating contacts between technologies and patients. This includes collecting information from patients, assessing a patient's health condition based on biodata provided by telemonitoring devices and their own experiential knowledge, instructing patients on how to use the telemonitoring devices, and entering data into the electronic data systems. Moreover, telecare workers act as intermediaries among technologies, patients and traditional healthcare professionals. This intermediary work includes informing the attending healthcare professionals about the results of telemonitoring, that is, assessment of ECGs, weight or blood pressure, and contacting them to ask for medical interventions such as changing medication or admission to hospitals. The work of telecare professionals is, however, not restricted to these more or less instrumental tasks. A substantial portion of telecare work consists of filling the gaps between the scripts of the various technical devices, setting patients' minds at ease, and social talk with patients. I described how telecare professionals are important actors in managing the consequences of the distributed nature of the work involved in diagnosing and monitoring the bodies of actors who are geographically separated. Although this articulation work and affective work is absent in dominant discourses on telecare technologies, for patients it makes all the difference. Telecare workers enable patients to build trust in the new technology and to adopt the tasks and responsibilities delegated to them in the geography of telecare.

This conclusion is not restricted to the telecare devices described in this book. In their study of telecare technologies designed to support frail, elderly people in order that they may remain living at home in the UK, Celia Roberts and Maggie Mort emphasize the importance of the communication skills and emotional work of call centre operators in providing care for these older people (Roberts and Mort, 2009).

Despite their crucial role, telecare workers do not have an easy life. Their professional identity can best be described as being caught between the scripts of technical devices, norms of care, and the boundary work of the established medical professions. My analysis shows how telecare work largely depends on, and is defined by, various technical devices. The scripts of telemonitoring devices, the phone, and electronic triage systems constitute telecare work as highly pre-structured and protocol-driven. The healthcare professional created in telemedical centres is disciplined to prioritize the objective, standardized knowledge scripted in technological devices over their own practical knowledge. Fortunately, there are escape routes. Although ICT-based technologies impose a structure upon telecare providers' work, the technical devices included in telecare technologies are not equally influential in pre-structuring and defining this work. Of the technological devices that constitute telecare technologies, the telemonitoring system (in Germany and the Netherlands) and the electronic triage system (in the Netherlands) have the most compulsory scripts. Both systems force actions upon telenurses in such a way that they cannot escape the script for collecting and entering data. The phone, as representative of the generation of communication technologies prior to the introduction of ICT-based communication technologies, grants more responsibility and control to telecare workers than the new communication technologies, that is, telemonitoring and the electronic triage system. The ways in which technologies structure the work of telecare professionals thus illustrates how technologies that consist of multiple devices may give more flexibility to users who can bypass the script of one particular device because they can rely on the scripts of other devices. In my account, the old-fashioned phone thus emerges as an important technology that enables telecare professionals to work around parts of the scripts of the ICT-based devices in the telemedical centre. The use of the phone enables them to build on and extend their practical knowledge. My analysis shows how telecare workers continue to value their own expertise and tacit knowledge: they do not passively follow the actions scripted in the digital devices but rely on their practical knowledge. As other sociologists of medicine and technology have argued, healthcare work cannot be entirely captured in protocols and standards because it involves interpretation and inter-subjectivity. Interactions between nurses and patients are based on interpretation in which experiential and tacit knowledge are crucial (Berg, 1997; Hanlon, 2005). The reliance on practical knowledge can thus be understood as an important, although often implicit, strategy of telecare workers to ensure that the care they deliver remotely meets their own standards.

In addition to technical devices and norms of care, the professional identity of telecare providers is also defined by the boundary work of the established medical professions. Telecare workers as newcomers in the medical world were not exactly welcomed with open arms, to put it mildly. As we have seen, the boundary work of traditional healthcare professionals resulted in a situation in which telecare work became restricted to advisory work. Medical interventions, that is, changing medication and producing diagnoses, remained in the hands of cardiologists, general practitioners, and heart-failure nurses. Telecare workers are expected to provide services to, and support the work of, traditional healthcare practitioners. The geography of telecare thus involves a distribution of labour based on a hierarchical relationship between telecare and traditional healthcare professionals. In this emerging landscape of care, gender is also implicated. By employing women as telenurses and men as telephysicians and supervisors, the German centre, and to a lesser extent the Dutch centre, built on and reinforced the gendered hierarchy of labour that still dominates the healthcare sector in many countries. These gender politics are not restricted to the telecare centres in Germany and the Netherlands. In their study of telecare technologies for frail, elderly people in the UK, Roberts and Mort observed that the workers in the telecall centres are mainly women (Roberts and Mort, 2009, p. 144).

A second major group implicated in the geography of responsibilities inscribed in telecare technologies whose work is largely absent in dominant discourses of the new technology is patients. As described in the previous chapters, telecare devices delegate specific tasks and responsibilities for diagnosing and monitoring heart problems to patients. Because of the introduction of the ambulatory ECG-recorder, the heart mobile phone and the heart-failure monitoring system, producing ECGs or measuring weight or blood pressure is no longer restricted to health-care professionals. Telecare technologies thus contribute to redefining the identities of patients. Instead of being passive recipients of health-care, patients are expected to act as diagnostic agents or inspectors of their own bodies. The work delegated to patients thus goes far beyond the instrumental tasks described in the promises on telecare producers' websites for patients. Patients are expected not only to use a technical device but also to diagnose and monitor heart diseases in the absence of healthcare professionals. This dual task of mastering a technology and diagnosing and monitoring bodies makes the work of patients much harder and more consequential than the work involved in domesticating consumer technologies for entertainment and leisure, technologies frequently studied by scholars in cultural and media studies.

My analysis of the work and responsibilities delegated to patients also shows a third subject position for patients: patients as producers of biodata. Heart patients are expected to play an active role in producing more and more data that travel through an extensive network of telemedical centres, hospitals, general practitioners' rooms, health-insurance companies, and clinical research departments. Patients are expected to make their bodies available and accessible not just to their own family doctors, cardiologists or heart-failure nurses, but also to a whole, materially connected, network of people and organizations they will never visit or meet in person. This subject position of patients enables telecare technologies to act as 'witness-producing machines', to use the term Jette Aroe Clausen introduced to refer to electronic foetal monitoring systems (Clausen, 2008). Equally importantly, the active involvement of patients in diagnosing and monitoring heart diseases extends the clinical gaze to non-professionals. In the geography of telecare, patients no longer yield the inspection of their bodies solely to healthcare professionals. This change in the tasks and responsibilities of patients introduces other ways of knowing bodies. Similarly to what sociologists of technology have described for self-care technologies, telecare devices contribute to objectifying the body and providing other knowledge than patients' own subjective experience of health and illness (Prout, 1996; Langstrup Nielsen, 2003). In addition to causing health problems or pain, bodies become a source of objectified, medical knowledge, not only for doctors but also for patients.

Reflecting on these different identities ascribed to patients, we can conclude that telecare technologies introduce new forms of medical surveillance of bodies that require a rethinking of Foucauldian approaches to medicalization. Whereas Foucault (1973) described practices in medicine in which the medical gaze was restricted to healthcare professionals, and patients subjected their bodies to medical inspection, telecare technologies constitute bodies that are scrutinized not only by medical experts but also by patients and their partners at home. Telecare technologies thus extend the clinical gaze to patients and to non-clinical spaces. As other STS scholars have suggested, the surveillance of telecare technologies is no longer tied to the physical location of a panopticon-like clinic, which seems to suggest a de-centring of the clinical gaze (Mort et al., 2003; Langstrup Nielsen, 2003; Brown and Webster, 2004; Dubbeld, 2005). However, my analysis shows that there is more at stake. Telecare devices for heart patients participate in producing various kinds of surveillance processes that differ in agency and responsibilities delegated to patients. The heart mobile phone and the ambulatory ECG recorder constitute surveillance practices in which a large part of the responsibility is delegated to patients. Patients decide when and where to inspect their bodies, a process that is only marginally controlled by healthcare professionals or technical devices. In contrast, the heart-failure monitoring system introduces a more centralized form of surveillance in which telecare workers and technical devices exercise disciplinary power over patients. Although patients carry out the measurements themselves, the telemonitoring system and telenurses 'stand in' for control over their weight and blood pressure, taking away part of the responsibility from patients. Patients remain responsible for measuring weight and blood pressure and adhering to the bodily regime of medication, diet and exercise, but the control and interpretation of their bodily data is delegated to the system and healthcare professionals. This is in sharp contrast to the promises articulated by the producer of this telecare device that portray patients as 'managers of their own disease' or talk about empowering patients, which would suggest a redistribution of power between patients and healthcare professionals in which patients are more in control of guarding their health condition and interacting with healthcare professionals.

Telecare devices for heart patients thus produce a relationship between body and self in which the technology creates a form of patient 'who continues to be acted upon' (May et al., 2007), although there are differences in the degree of agency and responsibility granted to patients.

The participation of patients in telecare practices can thus be considered a double-edged sword. On the one hand, patients are made more active in gazing into their body, through which they become more knowledgeable about their own condition, which may contribute to their expertise. On the other hand, the system allows patients to learn more about their bodies and take action only within a set of predefined guidelines which delegates responsibilities and control largely to healthcare professionals and technical devices. I therefore conclude that telecare technologies not only participate in de-centring the clinic but also in re-centring the clinic. This re-centring of the clinical gaze is further reinforced because telecare devices help patients to refer the ownership of the bodily data collected by them and telecare devices to the digital database used by the healthcare professionals and health insurers who own and run the telemedical centres.

We thus can conclude that, although some acts of care and responsibilities are delegated to telecare workers, patients, and technical devices, control over this distributed clinical gaze remains firmly in the hands of the established medical professions, that is, cardiologists and general practitioners. This finding confirms studies of telecare technologies aimed at supporting independent living for elderly people, which emphasize that the transfer of care from hospitals and other institutional care settings to the home does not imply the demise of the traditional healthcare institutions (Milligan, 2009). Although telecare technologies can be considered as 'technologies of deinstitutionalization' (Mort et al., 2009, p. 11) by enabling care outside the traditional healthcare institutions, the control over care remains executed by these institutions. This centralized form of medical surveillance is even extended and reinforced because of the growing importance of health insurers and the emergence of telecare workers as respectively major and new actors in the changing landscape of healthcare. Although telecare technologies have the potential, and were meant to bypass and partly replace traditional healthcare professionals and institutions, telecare technologies adapt to rather than transform the established hierarchy in the order of who cares. Owing to the boundary work of general practitioners, cardiologists, and heart-failure nurses, two of the three telecare devices featured in this book were redesigned to accommodate resistance from the established medical professions. As we have seen, the resistance of general practitioners to the heart mobile phone resulted in a redesign of the device to enable a shift in primary users from patients to general practitioners. The case of the heart-failure telemonitoring system showed a similar pattern, although resistance was not so much directed to the telecare system as to the telemedical centre that acted as intermediary between healthcare professionals and patients. The inter-professional competition among cardiologists, heart-failure nurses, and telecare professionals eventually resulted in a repositioning of the telecare system in the landscape of healthcare.

Instead of introducing the telemedical centre as an obligatory point of passage to the telecare system, the technology was put on the market as a system that also could be used by directly sending patients' data to the heart-failure polyclinic. In this way, cardiologists and heart-failure nurses could keep the care of patients in their own hands.

My account of telecare technologies for heart patients thus shows how the distribution of responsibilities inscribed in telecare devices clashed with the pre-existing distribution of responsibilities and power. This clash resulted in a geography of care which grants more responsibility and control to the established medical professions than to telecare workers and patients.

How places matter: The changing spatial dimensions of healthcare

Although the established healthcare professionals have been successful in guarding the hierarchy of the order of care, this does not mean that healthcare has remained largely untouched when telecare devices have been introduced. As I described in the previous chapters, the implementation and use of telecare technologies imply a transformation of the landscape of healthcare in which care becomes geographically dispersed over already established places, but also over new spaces where acts of care take place. Compared to other healthcare practices, geographical distance is thus integral to telecare.

Telecare technologies affect distance and place in a double sense. On the one hand, they create distances because they introduce a situation in which acts of care take place while patients and healthcare providers are geographically separated. On the other hand, telecare devices aim to erase distances by introducing virtual encounters between patients and healthcare professionals. Patients no longer have to visit the doctor frequently, and vice versa, because interactions are mediated by ICT-based devices. This does not mean that places are no longer important. In this book, I have attempted to provide a critical intervention into discourses that celebrate the erasure of distance and place by ICT-based devices. The techno-geographical approach introduced in this book has enabled me to show how places still matter. A focus on geography provided an appropriate heuristic by which to study the co-construction of technologies and places. In this respect the network metaphor, often used by STS scholars, is problematic because networks are non-geographical by definition, thus neglecting the importance of place (Henke and Gieryn, 2008). In contrast, the technogeographical approach emphasizes the place-dependency of the interrelationships between people and technologies.

This book shows four different ways in which telecare technologies transform the spatial dimensions of healthcare:

1 Telecare technologies change the geography of healthcare by introducing telecare centres as new spaces of care, a process discussed in the previous section of this chapter.
2 Telecare technologies contribute to redefining familiar places, most notably the home and public places, into spaces of care. In this process, the experience and meaning of these spaces also changes.
3 Spaces in which telecare technologies are introduced shape the use and meaning of these devices, which underscores the place-dependency of user–technology relations.
4 Telecare technologies participate in creating virtual spaces that introduce new forms of care based on digital proximity, resulting in specific technologies of self.

Let me first summarize and reflect on how telecare technologies affect the home and public spaces. My analysis shows how the home is no longer the same when it becomes electronically connected with and morally integrated into the broader landscape of healthcare, including telemedical centres, hospitals, and general practitioners' offices. In contrast to the dominant discourses on telecare technologies, which portray patients' homes as a tabula rasa, I described how telecare devices cannot simply be inserted into the home without changing the lived experiences in and meanings of places we call home. Ambulatory ECG-recorders, electronic blood pressure meters, and scales as new inhabitants of the home intervene drastically and change daily routines and social relationships within the home. The example of the heart-failure telemonitoring system illustrates how the introduction of this new technology in the home challenges daily routines because it involves much more that just using a medical device for a couple of minutes a day, as the producer of this telecare device for heart-failure patients promised potential users. The use of the heart-failure telemonitoring device implies a transgression of the boundaries between the home and the clinic. This telecare device transforms the home from a private place into a hybrid space where private and public spheres become closely intertwined and redefined. In this 'home-hospital hybrid' (Willems, 2008), patients have to change their daily routines at home by making their bodies accessible to remote healthcare providers by measuring and sending key diagnostic markers of their disease daily at a more or less fixed moment of the day. Equally importantly, they have to be available to healthcare professionals for feedback on their measurements and health conditions. As we have seen, this continuous availability changes practices and the meaning of time spent at home. A morning ritual with telecare devices is definitely different from waking up and enjoying your breakfast without having to measure your blood pressure and weight. Similarly, being in control over time throughout the day creates a different experience of home than a day interrupted by flashing lights from a set-top box or phone calls from telenurses. As Dick Willems has suggested, we may wonder 'what remains of the home as the private area *par excellence* when it takes on at least some characteristics of the hospital, an almost public space' (Willems, 2008, p. 63). The ways in which the telecare technologies transform the home are not restricted to the devices described in this book. In their discussion of telecare devices for disabled and elderly people, Christine Milligan and colleagues emphasize that these care technologies act to 'circumvent "the door"', opening up new ways of entering the home and enabling care professionals 'to "appear" in the home albeit without physical presence'. They portray these technologies as actors that create 'cracks in the door' (Milligan et al., 2010, p. 34).

The telecare technology for heart-failure patients thus participates in a transformation in which patients' homes become attuned to the routines of the clinic. This change affects not only patients but also other inhabitants of the home, particularly the partners of patients. As I described, partners are turned into co-inspectors of patients' bodies. They are actively engaged in watching graphs on TV, paying attention to the signals of the telemonitoring system, and even sometimes taking over these tasks and responsibilities from their partners. This telecare device thus participates in transforming the inspection of bodies into a collective endeavour of telecare devices, telenurses, cardiologists, patients, and their partners.

As we have seen, gender is also implicated. The involvement of partners in using telecare devices shows important gender dynamics. Although telecare devices act as gender benders by delegating responsibilities for taking care of health problems to both women and men, thus disrupting a traditional gendered division of care, my analysis of use practices illustrates how men and women tend to adhere to a gendered distribution of responsibilities at home where men do the technical and women the emotional work.

Most importantly, this transformation of the home into an electronic outpost of the clinic was not embraced by all patients. As we have seen, some patients refused to take the clinic home. Heart-failure patients thus definitely do not all share the same perception of the new technology. Whereas some patients are very willing to integrate this telecare device into their daily lives, others consider the new technology as an unwelcome intruder into their homes and lives. These voluntary non-users actively defended the boundaries between home and clinic because they valued their freedom and independence at home. My analysis of the ambulatory ECG recorder shows similar dynamics of how telecare devices affect patients' homes. Although the script of this technology introduces a less strict regime of accessibility and availability of bodies, that is, patients are allowed to choose the moment to register and send ECGs themselves, so more responsibility and control are delegated to patients, the use of the ambulatory ECG-recorder definitely changes the patient's experience of being at home. As I described, this telecare device disturbs their sleep at night, changes the ways in which they have to use their phones, makes them anxious about when to make an ECG, and creates a constant awareness of their heart problem.

Telecare technologies not only contribute to redefining the home; they also participate in changing public places into spaces of care. In this book, public spaces emerged as a second important place that matters in telecare. The use of the ambulatory ECG-recorder outside the home exemplifies how this telecare device redefines patients' presence in, and experience of public spaces. Shopping malls and trains turn into potentially threatening places because the beeping sound of the telecare device can attract the attention of others and lead to an involuntary disclosure of patients' heart problems to strangers. As we have seen, many patients considered the sound of this telecare device as an undesirable transgression of the boundaries between their public and private lives. They resisted this indiscretion of the new technology by inventing new ways to carry the ambulatory ECG-recorder with them in order to regain control over the agency of the device. Other patients decided not to use this telecare technology outdoors to avoid any violation of their privacy. We thus can conclude that the redefinition of public places as spaces of care is not unproblematic, an issue I return to in the last section of this chapter.

Virtual encounters: Telecare technologies as compulsory technologies of self

My techno-geographical account of telecare technologies shows not only how telecare technologies transform familiar places such as the home and public places into new spaces of care that shape the meaning and use of technical devices. As described briefly above, the focus on geography is also important to understanding how the new technology redefines the spatial dimensions of healthcare by introducing virtual encounters between healthcare professionals and patients. Telecare devices imply a move in healthcare from physical places such as hospitals, policlinics and general practitioners' consulting rooms to telemediated care. In this book I described this transformation as a shift from healthcare based on face-to-face contacts to a new form of care in which interactions between healthcare professionals and patients rely on digital proximity. As we have seen, telecare technologies drastically challenge long-established forms of proximity between healthcare providers and patients in which doctors and nurses could physically touch and care for patients. What sets telecare apart from face-to-face care is that it is provided by a new collective of technical devices, telecare professionals, and patients whose members are not in the same place. Some of the technical devices are in patients' homes (recorders, scales, meters, set-top boxes, TVs and phones), whereas others are located in telemedical centres (telemonitoring and electronic triage systems, phones, and electronic data-storing systems) or invisibly present outdoors (satellites, copper wires and glass fibres). Most importantly, patients and telecare professionals are very definitely spatially separated: they will never meet one another in real life. The kind of care provided by this spatially separated, but materially connected, collective can be characterized by two interrelated dimensions:

1 Telecare disciplines patients to inspect their bodies at home and in public spaces continuously by acts of care inscribed in technical devices.
2 Telecare defines disorders and bodies in terms of hard numbers.

To be sure, dimensions of telecare should not be considered as intrinsic capacities of telecare technologies. However, the three devices investigated in this book show similarities that illustrate how telecare for heart patients differs from face-to-face care. Let me first reflect on how telecare technologies operate as disciplinary technologies. A major difference between diagnostic and monitoring procedures based on physical and virtual encounters is that the inspection of bodies is no longer an isolated, individual act that patients can perform wherever and whenever they prefer. Instead, the inspection of bodies is turned into a collective endeavour of patients, telecare devices, telecare professionals, and traditional healthcare providers. In this collective, some actors are more important than others. As we have seen, the three technical devices participate in constituting different geographies of telecare in which some devices (the ambulatory ECG-recorder and the cardiophone) grant more agency and responsibility to patients than the other telecare device (the heart-failure monitoring system). Despite these differences, all devices are involved in creating virtual encounters between healthcare providers and patients which redefine the diagnostic and monitoring practices of heart patients into daily, continuous medical surveillance. This is a major difference from similar healthcare provisions that take place during physical encounters, which constitute the surveillance of bodies as an intermittent process. Although surveillance based on face-to-face contacts between healthcare professionals and patients also follows specific procedures, they may vary in the frequency of visits to policlinics and general practitioners' offices, the personal routines of patients' keeping diaries of measurements, and patients' initiatives to contact healthcare professionals based on their own subjective experience of heart problems. These monitoring practices can thus be considered as rather flexible forms of disciplining bodies. In contrast, surveillance based on virtual encounters requires an 'immediate form of presence and agency' of patients (Finch et al., 2006) and introduces very explicit and forceful scripts for collaboration and interdependencies between patients and healthcare professionals. Consequently, telecare introduces rather rigid forms of disciplining bodies.

As I have argued in Chapter 8, the different ways in which telecare and face-to-face care discipline bodies can best be understood by using Foucault's notion of technologies of self. Telecare technologies participate in introducing specific technologies of self in which taking care of oneself is transformed into a compulsory rather than a voluntary act. The ways in which telecare devices act as technologies of self are relevant to debates on responsibility and self-care. Since the 1990s, encouraging patients to take more responsibility for their own health has been considered as crucial in dealing with the chronic illnesses of late modern society, a view articulated by public health agencies such as the World Health Organization. In these debates, telecare is usually portrayed as a technology that 'increases the potential for patients to take on more responsibility for their health care' (Kendall, 2001). My analysis indicates that telecare technologies for heart patients do not fulfil this promise: they delegate responsibilities and control largely to technological devices and medical experts rather than to patients. Reflecting on the concept of self-care, which has a double meaning, namely caring for oneself and by oneself, we can conclude that tele-monitoring technologies constitute self-care primarily as care for one-self and not so much by oneself. In contrast, diagnostic and monitoring practices based on face-to-face contacts constitute self-care as both car-ing for yourself and by yourself. Moreover, it constitutes self-care as a voluntary rather than a compulsory act. Patients themselves determine how, where and when they monitor their bodies and whether they think it is necessary to call for assistance from medical experts. They also retain the ownership of their bodily data, thus escaping continuous surveillance by medical experts.

A second way in which healthcare based on virtual encounters differs from face-to-face care is in the diagnosis and monitoring of diseases being restricted to 'hard numbers' (Moser, 2008, p. 73). As Ingunn Moser has described for telecare technologies for the elderly, the telecare devices described in this book favour hard numbers on heart activity, blood pressure, and body weight which stand in for the health condi-tion of heart patients. Telecare thus introduces very specific forms of technologies of self in which taking care of your heart is transformed into measuring ECGs, blood pressure, or weight. Telecare systems allow patients to learn more about their bodies and take action within a set of predefined guidelines, which constitute patients' bodies as standard-ized. In this process of standardization, measurements for weight, blood pressure, and ECGs become the norm. Knowing bodies and coping with disease at home is thus no longer restricted to patients' subjective experience of health and illness but is also shaped by figures represent-ing vital signs. Although diagnostic and monitoring practices based on face-to-face care also rely increasingly on standardized representations of key diagnostic markers, the awareness and treatment of heart prob-lems as diseases that can be controlled by taking care of your weight, blood pressure, or ECG becomes more powerful when it is embedded in a telecare system that disciplines patients to check these vital signs daily than when it only features in conversations with the attending physi-cian, in laboratory results, or in information leaflets.

Equally importantly, the reliance on hard numbers as representa-tives of the health condition of heart patients neglects other relevant medical indictors, such as skin colour, breathing problems, or swollen legs, as well as psychosocial aspects and patients' own accounts of how they feel. This is clearly illustrated in my comparison of face-to-face with telecare for heart-failure patients. Whereas nurses in policlinics included observations of skin colour and the condition of patients' legs and breath into their accounts, and care for psychosocial problems was a crucial part of the care provided in the heart-failure policlinic, telecare prioritized a narrowly defined set of medical indicators of patients' conditions, although telenurses did their best to escape the scripts of the technology. As we have seen, in virtual encounters heart failure became constituted as a disease rather than an illness.

I therefore conclude that the healthcare provided in virtual encounters contributes to the biomedicalization of daily life. The term 'biomedicalization' has been introduced by Adele Clarke and her colleagues to refer to processes in which medicalization is reconstituted and extended through the introduction of new biomedical technologies, including genomics, transplant medicine, biotechnologies, and molecular biology. Biomedicalization differs from medicalization because it transforms medical phenomena rather than just exercising control over disorders or failing bodies (Clarke et al., 2003; Clarke et al., 2010). Actually, telecare technologies facilitate both processes. Telemediated care extends control over heart problems by drawing patients and their partners, telecare devices, and a whole new category of healthcare professionals and organizations as well as patients' homes and public spaces into the medical surveillance of heart problems. This intensified medicalization involves not only an increase in the actors, devices, and places involved in inspecting bodies; it also includes a change in scale. Telecare technologies drastically extend medicalization processes because they are targeted at the diagnosis and monitoring of diseases that occur frequently in Western industrialized countries, in this case heart rhythm irregularities and heart failure.

Telecare technologies thus clearly contribute to the medicalization of heart problems. However, the shift towards telemediated care also implies a biomedicalization. Telecare devices contribute to transforming heart diseases into a narrowly defined set of medical indicators, which redefine how heart diseases are diagnosed and monitored and what it means to be a heart patient. The introduction of surveillance practices based on virtual encounters between healthcare professionals and patients can thus be considered as a digital biomedicalization of daily life.

Desirable futures

The techno-geographical approach developed in this book is not only relevant to scholars and healthcare professionals who share an interest in the ways in which technologies transform healthcare. This approach is also relevant to designers and policymakers because it makes us sensitive to some critical issues concerning the future development of telecare technologies.

Drawing on the major findings of this book, I suggest that there are three decisive issues at stake. The first issue that requires careful consideration in the future development of telecare technologies is the place-dependency of the use and meaning of technical devices. An important insight of this study is that the same technological device can do different things in different places. My analysis of use practices of the ambulatory ECG-recorder illustrates how the small device changes from a more or less handy tool to diagnose heart-rhythm problems into a disrupter of the privacy of patients as soon as patients leave their homes and go shopping, to work, or to visit friends. In spaces outside the home, the telecare device turns into an indiscreet technology that transgresses the boundaries between the public and the private by making patients' heart problems audible and visible to others. What a technology means and how it is used (or not!) thus depends on the places where it is meant to be used. This place-dependency of the use and meaning of telecare devices has important consequences for the design and implementation of the new generation of telecare devices. Currently, one major focus in the design of telecare technologies is to develop devices that patients can use when they are on the move. The European Commission has funded R&D projects with telling names such as MobiHealth[1] which include the development of telecare systems consisting of sensors integrated in clothing worn on the body and devices that can be inserted inside the body that enable the measurement and sending of biodata from places outside the home. Although the promises articulated by designers and producers of the new generation of telecare devices emphasize that the mobility of these devices may improve the quality of care and quality of life, the research presented in this book tells a more complicated story. As we have seen, the use of telecare devices in public spaces complicates the lives of their users. Patients often develop careful strategies to keep others from discovering that something is wrong with their bodies. Although the beeping sounds of ICT gadgets are part and parcel of public spaces, the presence of beeps, or other feedback signals, of medical devices is far more sensitive because they can disclose information considered by many people as private. If design strategies for mobile telecare devices do not take into account the privacy problems related to using telecare systems in public spaces, they will run the risk that patients will use these devices only at home, which undermines the very aim of this new generation of telecare technologies.

A second important issue for the future development of telecare technologies is the kind of proximity between healthcare professionals and patients inscribed in telecare devices. My analysis shows the importance of socio-technical configurations that support specific forms of digital proximity. One of the major implications of implementing telecare technologies is that they replace the physical nearness of healthcare professionals to patients with an often asymmetrical digital proximity. Reflecting on the use practices of the ambulatory ECG-recorder and the heart-failure monitoring system, I conclude that two actors are of crucial importance to creating forms of digital proximity that support patients to become active participants in the diagnosis and monitoring of heart diseases: telecare workers and the telephone.

As we have seen, telecare professionals turned out to be of crucial importance, not only to reading and interpreting biodata and giving feedback to patients, but also to enabling patients to learn to use the telecare devices, to building trust in the new technology, to reducing their anxieties, and for social talk. Articulation and affective work can thus be considered as indispensable because they support forms of digital proximity that enable intimacy at a distance and decrease the risk of selective use or non-use.

This invisible work of telecare professionals is highly dependent on a second, non-human actor: the phone. In my account of telecare technologies for heart patients, the phone emerged as an important actor because it enabled direct communication between healthcare professionals and patients. In contrast to the ICT-based devices, which support only protocol-driven communication, the phone facilitates open, two-directional communication between healthcare providers and patients. This communication tool not only plays an important role in helping patients to act as diagnostic agents or inspectors of their bodies; it also turns out to be an important asset in helping telecare workers provide care that meets their standards. As I described previously, communication by phone enables telecare professionals to work around the abstract rationality inscribed in the ICT-based systems that structure telecare. By talking and listening to patients' stories they could build on and extend their practical knowledge which they considered just as important in assessing the health condition of heart patients. A technology that enables open communication between care providers and patients can thus be considered as a key technology to make up for the reduction of illness to hard numbers inscribed in telecare devices. Whereas ICT-based devices deliver abstract, codified information on heart diseases, the telephone can be considered as a technology that supports patients' subjective experience as an important resource for diagnosing and monitoring bodies. Equally importantly, the phone is crucial because it supports the 'sociality' of telecare technologies (Moser, 2008, p. 73). The direct communication line and the flexible script of the phone enable patients and telecare professionals to build trusting, social relationships. As we have seen, telecare workers consider it important to 'get to know' their patients, whereas patients rely on phone contacts to learn to cope with their diseases and to build trust in the technology and the telecare professionals. This sociality mediated by the phone is important because it makes up for the absence of direct personal contacts between healthcare providers and patients that characterizes telecare.

Again, there is a tension between this conclusion and trends in the current and future design of telecare technologies. New directions in the design of telecare technologies involve a move not only towards developing mobile devices, but also towards fully automated systems which require no intervention from (tele)healthcare professionals. Feedback and instructions given to patients will be delegated to the technology itself. For several years, international R&D consortia consisting of leading electronic industries, hospitals, and university-based research departments have aimed to develop software that can analyse biodata collected by wireless sensors and provide feedback on the health condition of patients and their adherence to prescribed therapies automatically (Royal Philips Electronics, 2008). The geography of care inscribed in this future generation of telecare devices implies that the tasks and responsibilities delegated to telecare professionals will be completely delegated to technical devices. This erasure of human actors suggests that telecare technologies can provide care all by themselves. As Maggie Mort and colleagues have suggested already, 'technologies do not care, they support care' (Mort et al., 2008, p. 96). My analysis further substantiates this argument by showing how telecare devices can contribute to providing care only when they are integrated into a socio-technical configuration that enables meaningful interactions between healthcare professionals, patients, and technological objects. The new generation of telecare devices ignores important actors in these collectives of people and objects. As we have seen, telecare professionals and the phone are crucial players in this configuration because they act as intermediaries between patients and technical devices.

We may thus expect new problems to arise when the new generation of telecare devices no longer includes these actors. Who or what assists patients when they face problems in using telecare technologies when these are fully automated? Who or what supports patients and health-care professionals in the case of failure of computer databases or telecare devices? Who or what facilitates communication between healthcare providers and patients when all interactions are delegated to so-called intelligent sensors that only process information? Replacing humans and the familiar phone by fully automated systems implies that telecare will be further reduced to hard numbers, which neglects the importance of affective and social relations for providing healthcare at a distance.

This bypassing of telecare workers and phone-mediated contacts implies an important shift in the identity of telecare devices. Whereas the current generation of telecare devices can be characterized as those that support information exchange and communication (ICTs), fully automated systems are merely information technologies (ITs). In this respect, this trend in the development of telecare technologies differs from the development of ICT systems in other sectors (e.g. business and traffic) where there is more emphasis on communication or social media. This book clearly shows that a reduction of telecare devices to IT systems runs the risk of creating and using technologies that fail to support healthcare.

A third, and last, decisive issue for the future development of telecare technologies is the extent to which these technical devices are attuned to the diversity of patients. An important insight of this book is that the same technical device can do and mean different things to different people. Let me begin with the example of the ambulatory ECG-recorder. As we have seen, this telecare device participates in making patients active participants in producing diagnoses, but it does not work this way for all heart patients. Because of the sound script and the use of Dutch in instructing and communicating with patients, the ambulatory ECG-recorder could become a useful technology only for detecting heart-rhythm problems for people who do not have hearing deficiencies and can understand Dutch. People who do not meet these requirements inscribed in the telecare device – particularly (elderly) people with hearing problems and the older generation of immigrants in the Netherlands – face unanticipated problems in using this telecare device and are therefore excluded as potential users of the new technology. The role of language in building relationships of trust, both with healthcare professionals and towards technical devices, seems to be very important and becomes even more relevant in case telecare centres are moved to Asian countries or other countries with languages and cultures that differ from patients' backgrounds, as has happened with other ICT-based services (Milligan et al., 2010, p. 31).

The heart-failure monitoring system illustrates another way in which the same device can do and mean different things to different people. Whereas for some patients this telecare device became a reassuring technology ('the doctor is always with me'), for other patients the technology was a device that increased their anxiety and reinforced feelings of a failing body, or, for their partners, feelings of guilt. These patients, often women, refused to use the heart-failure monitoring system because they considered the technology an unwelcome intruder in their lives that disturbed their peace of mind and independence. My account of telecare devices for heart patients thus illustrates how the diversity of patients, including physical conditions, age, gender, ethnicity, and attitude to coping with disease, matter in shaping user-technology relations.

We can thus conclude that the same technical device has many different faces for patients, which has important implications for healthcare policy and design. Governmental and managerial policies that aim to empower patients to take an active role in healthcare, as telecare advocates promise, should be more sensitive to the view that the diversity of patients requires a diversity of technical devices and healthcare provisions. Although design strategies usually focus on standardizing technology which results in a standard package for all patients that is blind to difference, the heterogeneity and diversity of patients, in terms of physical capacities, demographic background, and embodied experiences with new technologies, require a design strategy that aims to develop a variety of technical devices, which may include different feedback systems, different languages, and different degrees in control and autonomy delegated to its users.

As we have seen, not all heart patients embrace the sort of life built into telecare technologies. The heart-failure patients who figured as non-users in this book are very much aware of how the new technology affects their daily lives and actively defend their privacy and reject the compulsory character of the monitoring device.

Sensitivity to the diversity among patients therefore also touches on normative concerns. Telecare devices are not neutral devices; they act as 'moral machines'.[2] The morality inscribed in telecare devices concerns a sort of life in which the daily inspection of bodies, disciplining patients to follow medical regimes, and transforming illness into hard numbers has become the norm. Design strategies that narrow the development of telecare technologies to developing devices that enforce a strict compliance with medical instructions and standards introduce forms of life in which non-compliance or alternative ways of monitoring and living with failing bodies become non-existent. These developments in telecare have triggered a debate among sociologists and policymakers about the limits of what technological systems are allowed to do in making patients more compliant and whether patients are still allowed to be non-compliant.[3] Design strategies that aim to develop telecare devices with more flexible and diverse scripts could learn from these debates by taking into account the various ways in which patients relate to medical regimes and standards.

My analysis of the heart-failure monitoring systems indicates that systems that are too compulsive may eventually not succeed in making patients more active in healthcare because they take away too much of their responsibility. Instead, telecare systems that are less coercive and put more trust in patients' and healthcare providers' practical knowledge and creativity may prove to be better tools for supporting patients who wish to play an active role in healthcare.[4]

Design strategies that anticipate these different approaches to healthcare and the different capacities and attitudes among patients become even more urgent when national or governmental health policies decide to replace existing face-to-face healthcare provisions with telecare technologies. As I described in the first chapter, the introduction of telecare technologies is related to a neo-liberal political agenda, which aims to modernize and rationalize healthcare, decrease costs, and increase the profits of healthcare. Controlling and decreasing healthcare spending is a major concern for healthcare insurers, government agencies, and managers of healthcare organizations in Western industrialized countries in order to reduce fears that the provision of healthcare is no longer affordable. In this political economy of healthcare it seems likely that increasing pressures will arise to restrict healthcare services to telecare that is considered more cost-effective than the alternative healthcare provisions based on face-to-face contacts between healthcare providers and patients. Moreover, a further neo-liberalization of healthcare implies that telecare systems are offered as commodities in a healthcare market, which is, as we have seen, problematic not only because patients do not seem to be willing to pay for telecare products themselves, but also because it denies access to telecare for those patients who cannot afford it.

This development is very problematic because it implies an increase in inequities in access to healthcare. What would happen to Mr X, the heart patient introduced in the beginning of this book? What happens to him, and to other patients who refuse to use, or have problems using, telecare devices when healthcare insurance policies force them to use telecare and no longer offer any alternatives? As recent studies indicate, patients worry increasingly about cutting down current healthcare provisions based on personal, face-to-face contacts with healthcare providers or changes in healthcare provision in which telecare is offered as 'all or nothing' (Mort et al., 2009, p. 23; Maltha et al., 2003; SCP, 2005). This concern was addressed also at a recent conference on telecare held in London (March 2011) and attended by major stakeholders from Europe and the US, where 'fear about loss of human contact' was mentioned as one of the reasons for the 'limited uptake' of telecare technologies (Mattke, 2011). This underlines my argument that telecare cannot and should not be considered as an alternative to face-to-face care; telecare does not replicate existing healthcare provisions, but introduces healthcare practices that implicate other patient and professionals identities and forms of care.

A desirable future for Mr X and other heart patients would be if the move towards empowering patients to play an active role in healthcare included the provision of telecare and face-to-face care as different, but equally important and affordable, forms of care.

Notes

Chapter 1

1. This scenario is based on an interview with a heart-failure patient who was invited to participate in the clinical testing of a telemonitoring system recently introduced in the Netherlands but resisted using the device. Currently, the health insurance company reimburses the costs of the telemonitoring system; one of the managers informed us that compulsory use of the system will be part of their future policy (Interview Boutkan and Helm, 2006).
2. Because of the variety of ICT applications available for health purposes, various names are given to this new technology, including telemedicine, tele(health)care, patient telemonitoring technology, and e-health. The use of these terms in the literature is, however, not consistent: different terms are often used to refer to the same technological device. In this book, I use the Cochrane definition that distinguishes telemedicine from telecare. Cochrane defines telemedical technology as devices that support remote interactions between healthcare professionals, whereas telecare technology refers to applications that enable remote contacts between healthcare professionals and patients (Currell, 2000). I use the term 'telecare technology' to refer to technological devices that support the diagnosis and monitoring of patients by means of information and communication technologies.
3. Lehoux, P., Sicotte, C., Denis, J.-L., Berg, M., Lacroix, A. 2002. "The theory of use behind telemedicine: how compatible with physicians' clinical routines?" *Social Science & Medicine* 54: 889–904.
4. Wahlberg et al., 2003, and Johnson Pettinari and Jessop, 2001 for an overview of the literature on telephone-based health services.
5. Interview Murin, 2005. The Dutch health insurer Achmea faced strong resistance when they first introduced a phone-based service to support general practitioners. Owing to resistance from general practitioners, the health insurer not only terminated this service but also changed the name of their centre from medical call centre to medical service centre.
6. For an overview of research on the dynamics of user–technology relations, see Oudshoorn and Pinch, 2007.
7. I use the term traditional healthcare professionals to distinguish healthcare professionals, who provide face-to-face care, from telecare professionals, who deliver healthcare remotely.
8. Compared to the US, healthcare organizations in Europe are still predominantly located in the public sector, although there is a trend towards the privatization of healthcare, which is discussed below.
9. See Balka et al., 2009 for a more extensive discussion of the complex relationships between gender, healthcare and technologies.
10. See Mol, 2008 for a critical analysis of the emphasis on free choice by patients in these discourses.

11. This situation may change in the near future because of the new healthcare policy of the Obama administration since 2009.

Chapter 2

1. The term 'material-semiotic' was coined by Donna Haraway (1991). She introduced the term to refer to the complex, multiple ways in which materiality and meanings are inextricably intertwined.
2. For detailed analyses of how new health technologies transform human lives, see Berg and Mol, 1998; Brown and Webster, 2004; Webster, 2006 and 2007; Lehoux, 2006; Oudshoorn and Pinch, 2003; Timmermans and Berg, 2003; Mol, 2002 and 2008.
3. To be sure, the relevance of including place in studying science and technology has also been articulated by several scholars in the field of science and technology studies. This renewed interest in place is related to the rather bold claim that places are no longer relevant because, owing to the emergence of Internet, we live in a 'network society' characterized by a compression of space and time (Castells, 2000; Harvey, 1990; Cairncross, 1997; Kolko, 2000). In the *Handbook of Science and Technology Studies* (2008), Christopher Henke and Thomas Gieryn challenged this view by describing how spaces still matter in science. In their criticism, they also included actor network theory (ANT), because this approach puts to much emphasis on 'the mobility or flows of heterogeneous actants through networks ... thereby diminishing the apparent significance of the specific geographical places where the actants pass through or end up' (Henke and Gieryn, 2008, p. 354). Reflecting on previous and current research in science and technology studies, they emphasize how the very places in which scientific enquiry is situated, including laboratories, field sites, and museums, shape the production of scientific knowledge and practices and contribute to the credibility of knowledge claims. 'Science has a geography,' as Thomas Gieryn claimed as early as in the late 1990s (Gieryn, 1998, p. 248; Gieryn, 2006, p. 5), an argument elaborated on by David Livingstone in his book with the telling title *Putting Science in Its Place* (2003). The debate on the importance of place is not restricted to studies on science but also includes technologies. An exemplary study in this respect is Glen Norcliffe's attempt to extend and refine the social construction of technology approach (SCOT) to pay more attention to the geographical settings in which technological innovation occurs (Norcliffe, 2009). Reflecting on these studies, we can conclude that they primarily focus on the production of scientific knowledge and technological artifacts. As such, this body of literature thus reflects a tendency in STS to prioritize production over use, a position that has long been criticized by many scholars (Oudshoorn and Pinch, 2003 and 2007). My research aims to contribute to the ongoing debate on the importance of place by including use practices of technology in the analysis.
4. See Poland et al. 2005 for a discussion of the different approaches in health geography towards the role of place and space in health and social care.

In this paper, the authors describe the shift in this field from a narrow conceptualization of space as a 'geometric variable', which dominated early health geography (1960–90), towards a broader conceptualization. In this paper they introduce the notion of 'culture of place' to capture the complex interactions between culture, place, technology, and power.

5. Although Madeleine Akrich also included the importance of place to understand user–technology relationships, her interest was primarily in how engineers anticipate and define the places in which technologies are supposed to be used.

6. The choice of this term is inspired by the work of Flis Henwood and colleagues, who introduced the concept of 'technobiographies' to refer to the role of technologies in people's daily lives and the implicated different techno-social relationships (Henwood et al., 2001; Kennedy, 2003).

7. Actually, Roger Silverstone and colleagues were among the first scholars to draw attention to the relationships between technology and the home. In their influential work on domestication theory, they described how the home is an important place for 'taming' new technologies, a process in which social relations within the home and relations with friends and family are transformed (Silverstone and Haddon 1996; Silverstone and Hirsch, 1992). However, these studies did not address care technologies but focused primarily on consumer technologies.

8. This explanation was often articulated during my interviews with producers of telecare technologies.

9. Thanks to Wesley Shrum for mentioning this term.

10. Sally Wyatt identified four different types of non-user: 'resisters' (people who have never used the technology because they do not want to), 'rejecters' (people who no longer use the technology, because they find it boring or expensive or because they have alternatives), 'the excluded' (people who have never used the technology, because they cannot gain access for a variety of reasons), and 'the expelled' (people who stopped using the technology involuntarily because of cost or loss of institutional access) (Wyatt, 2003, p. 78).

11. The empirical data for this book are derived from a variety of sources. Chapter 3 is based on an analysis of websites of producers of telecare devices, press bulletins that announce the clinical testing and implementation of telecare devices, and brochures to promote the new technology among healthcare professionals in the US and Europe. Chapters 5, 7, and 8, are partly based on observations in telemedical centres in Germany and the Netherlands (including the Vitaphone Medical Service Centre in Chemnitz, Germany; the Achmea Medical Service Centre in Zwolle, the Netherlands; and the Hartis Telemedical Centre in Amsterdam, the Netherlands); a polyclinic for heart-failure patients at a Dutch hospital (the Medical Spectrum Twente, the main general hospital in Enschede, the Netherlands); and a Dutch home-care office in The Hague). In addition to observations, Chapters 7 and 8 are based on interviews with healthcare professionals and patients, and additional questionnaires completed by the latter. The empirical data for Chapter 7 were collected in the period April 2004 to February 2005. Interviews were held with managers of a Dutch company that provides cardiac telemonitoring services; a home-care office (responsible for

handing out ambulatory ECG-recorders and giving instructions to patients); and two general practitioners who prescribed ECG-recorders. In April and May 2004, a total of 95 patients made use of the telemonitoring system that we studied. Semi-structured, in-depth interviews were held with 11 of these patients. The remaining patient population received a questionnaire, 54 of which were returned. The empirical study presented in Chapter 8 was conducted in the period December 2005 to November 2007 and consisted of in-depth interviews and observations of five heart-failure patients who used a telemonitoring system during one year as part of a clinical trial and five patients who refused to participate in this trial. These patients relied on the monitoring service provided by heart-failure nurses at the polyclinic of the Medical Spectrum Twente, the main general hospital in Enschede, one of the five biggest cities in the Netherlands. Both users and non-users represented a variety of backgrounds in terms of demographics, disease history, and experience and attitude towards ICT devices. Finally, all the empirical chapters include information derived from interviews. Chapters 3, 4, and 5 draw on interviews with leading senior managers of firms in the telemedical industry in Germany and the Netherlands, a Dutch health insurance company, and a Dutch home-care organization (Chapter 1, 2, and 3). Chapters 4, 5, 6, 7, and 8 are based on interviews with general practitioners, clinicians, and nurses involved in the implementation and use of telecare devices for heart patients. The interviews and observations were conducted by Ivo Maathuis, a junior researcher, Lynsey Dubbeld, a post-doctoral researcher, and Nelly Oudshoorn.

Chapter 3

1. For a notable exception see Kornelia Konrad's study (2006) of expectation statements on electronic commerce and interactive television.
2. One notable exception is the study by Sturken et al., 2004. See also Abraham and Davis 2007, who argues that it is important to investigate later phases of the development of technologies to understand conflicting expectations, particularly around regulatory assessments.
3. Achmea and Philips. Press Information, 2005.
4. Achmea website, downloaded on November 24 2005. In the remaining references I will refer to this source as Achmea website, 2005.
5. Philips website, downloaded on November 25 2005. In the remaining references I refer to this source as Philips website, 2005.
6. In addition, Vitaphone has an extensive international network for the diffusion of its telecare products. Although most sales agents are located in Western European countries, the network also includes contacts with countries in Eastern Europe, Turkey, Greece, the US, China, India, and South Africa (website Vitaphone, downloaded February 9 2009).
7. Website Vitaphone (www.vitaphone.de), English version, downloaded 31 May 2006; Brochure Vitaphone downloaded from Vitaphone's website on 31 May 2006, pp. 5 and 10. In the remaining notes the first source is referred to as Website Vitaphone 2006, whereas the latter source is referred to as Brochure Vitaphone 2006.

8. Brochure Vitaphone, 2006.
9. Website Vitaphone, 2006. The GPS system of this version of the heart mobile phone could only be used outdoors. The later version of the heart mobile phone includes a so-called assisted GPS that can also locate people indoors as long as they are within 12 metres' reach of the outside (Interview Quinger, 2004).
10. The website analysed in this chapter was downloaded on 31 May 2006. More recently, Vitaphone has renewed its website. However, I have used the previous version because the website was in use during the period of my research when I conducted the interviews with staff and managers of Vitaphone in 2004. Although the new website adopts a different approach in addressing patients and healthcare professionals, most parts of the text are similar to those on the previous website. The text of the brochures has not been changed. The new version of the website is analysed in the next chapter because it reflects a strategy Vitaphone has adopted to solve the problems the company faced during the implementation of the heart mobile phone.
11. Website Vitaphone, 2006.
12. Website Vitaphone, 2006.
13. The new website of Vitaphone (downloaded on 8 January 2009) reflects this change. The text is no longer focused on Vitaphone's products but on the different heart diseases for which the telecare services are relevant. Viewers can no longer order a heart mobile phone by clicking on the website.
14. Website Vitaphone, 2006.
15. Brochure Vitaphone 2006, pp. 5 and 10.
16. Brochure Vitaphone 2006, pp. 14 and 15.
17. Brochure Vitaphone, 2006, p. 6.
18. Website Vitaphone, 2006.
19. Website Vitaphone, 2006.
20. Brochure Vitaphone, 2006, p. 13.
21. Website Vitaphone, 2006.
22. Brochure Vitaphone 2006, p. 12.
23. The later version of the website is different in this respect because it includes one link for patients and another link for medical professionals. (Website downloaded on 8 January 2009).
24. Brochure Vitaphone, 2006, pp. 5 and 14.
25. Brochure Vitaphone, 2006, p. 12.
26. Brochure Vitaphone, 2006, p. 12.
27. Website Vitaphone, 2006.
28. Brochure Vitaphone, 2006, p. 5.
29. Brochure Vitaphone, 2006, p. 5.
30. Website Vitaphone, 2006.
31. *Vitaphone 2300.* Brochure Vitaphone, 2006, p. 3.
32. Website Vitaphone, 2006.
33. Website Vitaphone, 2006.
34. Brochure Vitaphone, 2006, p. 8.
35. Brochure Vitaphone, 2006, p. 13.
36. Brochure Vitaphone, 2006, p. 13.
37. Website Vitaphone, 2006.
38. Brochure Vitaphone, 2006, p. 13.
39. Another name often used for this device is holterphone. This name refers to the forerunner of the ambulatory ECG-recorder: the holter, named after its

inventor Norman J. Holter. The holter is a portable device that can continuously monitor the electrical activity of the heart for between 24 and 48 hours. The first editions of the holter monitor used audio tapes to store the data, but since the 1970s digital memories have been used (diMarco et al., 1990: 53). The so-called 24-hour holter is used for ECG registration and evaluation, when patients with heart problems visit the cardiologist. The disadvantage of the holter is that it can be used for only one or two days, which reduces the chances of detecting heart-rhythm disturbances that often occur very infrequently. The ambulatory ECG-recorder aims to overcome this problem because it can monitor ECGs over a much longer period, usually a month. According to the director of Hartis, the portable ECG-recorder detects twice as many heart-rhythm disturbances as the 24-hour holter (Interview Holwerda, 2004).

40. Hartis website (www.hartis.nl) 28 November 2005 and downloaded on 13 April 2006. In the remaining notes this source will be referred to as Website Hartis, 2006.
41. Website Hartis, 2006. The way in which telecare devices are used in boundary work between healthcare professionals is discussed in the next chapter.
42. Website Hartis, 2006.
43. Website Hartis, 2006.
44. Website Vitaphone, English version (www.vitaphone.de), downloaded on 31 May 2006.
45. Website Hartis, 2006.
46. Website Hartis, 2006.
47. Website Hartis, 2006.
48. Website Hartis, 2006.
49. Remarkably, the promises of telecare technologies in Germany and the Netherlands do not include the argument that the new technology will improve access to healthcare for citizens who live in remote areas. This is in contrast to promises often articulated in other countries, such as Canada and the U.S. (Mort et al., 2003).
50. Although 'empowerment of patients' and 'patient compliance' are rooted in different discourses that take the perspective of the patient or the healthcare professional as referent, the promises articulated by Philips and Achmea do not make this distinction.

Chapter 4

1. In the past decade, both companies faced a rather disappointing diffusion of their telecare devices. Although Hartis's first director expected 60,000 patients to use the ambulatory ECG-recorder, the number of patients using the device rose to 6000 only in 2004 (Interview Holwerda, 2004). Vitaphone also failed to realize its promise to attract large numbers of users to its heart mobile phone as forecast by the US management consultants Frost & Sullivan, who expected that 'in Europe alone in 2011 over four million heart patients will own mobile devices that monitor their heart rates and are connected to a medical service' (Vitaphone brochure). By 2004, 800 people had bought a heart mobile phone and paid the monthly fee for the services of the telemedical centre (Interview Quinger, 2004).

2. Resistance to telecare devices developed by Philips was not restricted to the heart-failure telemonitoring system described in this chapter. Owing to resistance to earlier products, the company decided to halt previous attempts to introduce telecare technologies in Europe (Interview Quinger, 2004).

3. Inspired by Abbott, Thomas Gieryn (1983) introduced the concept of boundary work to refer to the processes underlying the demarcation of science from other social institutions or 'non-science'. In STS the concept of boundary work has subsequently been used to study the division of labour between science and policy, science and law and contests between scientific disciplines over disciplinary territory (Gieryn, 1983; Halffman, 2003).

4. Although the telecare device to diagnose heart-rhythm irregularities also faced resistance, I restrict my analysis to the telecare system for heart-failure patients and the heart mobile phone. The Hartis holterphone shows a dynamic in terms of resistance and boundary work similar to that of the heart mobile phone. As described in the previous chapter, Hartis performed boundary work by advertising the ambulatory ECG-recorder as a tool enabling general practitioners to remain active in the diagnosis of heart-rhythm disturbances, a field of expertise dominated largely by cardiologists.

5. Gatekeepers are those people who articulate and guard the boundaries of expert professions; the term was introduced by Crane, 1967.

6. Website Vitaphone, downloaded on 22 January 2009.

7. These differences in regulatory regime between medical devices and drugs do not mean that telecare firms do not try to get approval or a certificate for their healthcare products and services. In the US, Philips applied for and received marketing approval for the heart-failure telemonitoring system by the Food and Drug Administration (Interview Weijde, 2006). Vitaphone also applied successfully for quality assessment of its telecare services, not for the telecare devices but for its telemedical centre. In 2008, the Vitaphone Medical Service Centre received a certificate for the quality management system they had developed for implementing the services of the telemedical centre by the VDE Testing and Certification Institute in Germany. (Anonymous, 2008).

8. For privacy reasons I do not include the names of the heart-failure nurses.

9. The health insurer Achmea met resistance to their telemedical centre not only from cardiologists; they had similar experiences when they tried to introduce a tele-service to support general practitioners. The so-called general practitioner line was meant to reduce the workload of general practitioners by transferring patients' phone calls from the physician's rooms to telecare staff. The latter had to decide whether patients needed to visit the general practitioner or whether their problem could be solved by an advice by phone. This service of the telemedical centre, the same centre that runs the heart-failure telemonitoring system, was closed after two years because general practitioners did not want to collaborate any longer with the centre. (Anonymous, 2005).

Chapter 5

1. Exemplary studies that focus on traditional healthcare professionals include Cartwright, 2000; Mort et al., 2003; Bjorn and Balka, 2007. A notable exception

on the silencing of the work of telecare workers are the studies of Roberts and Mort (2009) and Milligan and colleagues (2010) on telecare devices for frail, elderly people that describe the work of telecare professionals at call centres in the UK.

2. The third telecare service investigated in this book is not included in this chapter because it is analysed in Chapter 8.

3. Actually, there is one male agent in the Chemnitz centre but he was not on duty during my visit (Interview Murin, 2005).

4. See Armstrong et al. 2007 for a discussion of the gendered nature of health-care work.

5. See Balka et al. 2009 for a detailed study of the changing relationships between gender and ICTs.

6. Because of high unemployment in Chemnitz, Vitaphone had no difficulty in hiring employees for its new centre. The job advertisements attracted more than 600 people, of whom 30 were eventually selected for the job (Interview Murin, 2005).

7. In Germany, half of the telenurses have no medical background, but graduated from university, received vocational training, or completed high school. The permanent staff of the centre consists of 24 agents, three supervisors, and two physicians. In addition, there are a couple of physicians-in-training affiliated with the hospital in Chemnitz, who work on a contract basis at the centre (Interview Murin, 2005). In the Netherlands, the medical service centre employs 50 part-time telenurses and three physicians. The service for heart-failure patients is run by four telenurses and one physician. (Interview Wal, 2006).

8. In the Netherlands the medical course was developed and taught by Hanneken Glazenburg, a heart-failure nurse affiliated with the MST hospital in Enschede (Interview Glazenburg, 2004). In Germany, the medical education programme was developed by Stefan Sack, the cardiologist who invented the heart mobile phone (Interview Sack 2004). Training of the staff in Chemnitz is conducted by one of the physicians, Dieter Wittig (Interview Wittig, 2005). The courses are followed by an examination (Interview Murin, 2005).

9. Two major exceptions are Michael 1996 and Kirejczyk 2000.

10. The TAS system is a slightly modified version of the electronic triage system used by the UK's National Health Service's health advice lines: NHS Direct. (Anonymous, 2002).

11. See Bjorn and Balka 2007 for a similar analysis of an electronic triage system in a Canadian hospital.

12. For a further analysis of the standardization and objectification of medical work see Suchman, 1994; Berg, 1997; Hanlon et al., 2005; Bjorn and Balka, 2007.

13. See Berg, 1997 for an exemplary study of how technological systems reinforce reductionist approaches to health.

14. See Hanlon, 2005, who made a similar argument in her study of an electronic triage system used in the UK NHS-Direct health advice lines.

15. For a similar analysis of the use of an electronic triage system in a Canadian hospital, see Bjorn and Balka, 2007.

16. ECG graphs of a 'normal' heart rhythm show a very regular pattern, whereas 'abnormal' heart rhythms will reveal a much less stable picture. According

to one of the German telephysicians, the skill to make a first assessment of ECGs can be rather easily acquired.
17. See, for example, Berg, 1997 and Hanlon, 2005.

Chapter 6

1. I focus only on physical and narrative proximity because moral proximity, 'in which nurses encounter the patient as other, recognise that a moral concern to "be for" exists, and are solicited to act on a patient's behalf' (Malone, 2003, p. 2318), is beyond the scope of this study.
2. Although both healthcare provisions have a similar aim, they reflect different approaches to resolving the tension between demand and resources in healthcare, described in the first chapter. Heart-failure policlinics represent a strategy that aims to reduce costs by delegating tasks and responsibilities from cardiologists to less expensive, specialized nurses. Telemonitoring technologies for heart-failure patients can be considered a more drastic strategy because care is delegated to a new healthcare infrastructure (the telemedical centre), a new category of healthcare staff (telenurses and telephysicians), and new technological devices.
3. Weight is an important indicator because a sudden increase in weight may be caused by the retention of fluid related to an increased dysfunction of the heart pump.
4. Although heart-failure patients who use the telemonitoring system also fill in questionnaires on their health condition, which include issues such as shortness of breath and swollen feet, telecare nurses did not mention these questionnaires as resources to provide healthcare remotely.
5. See Chapter 8 for an analysis of the role of patients' partners.

Chapter 7

1. In *Social Organization of Medicine*, Strauss and colleagues devoted one chapter examining the types of work patients do, how their work relates to the work of healthcare professionals, and how patients' work in hospital relates to their work at home. Although they refer to patients' work involved in using medical technologies, particularly kidney dialysis machines, they discuss this work primarily in terms of how it interferes with and differs from the work of healthcare professionals (Strauss et al., 1997, pp. 192, 201). I suggest that a focus on patient work is important as well to understanding all the (in)visible work involved in making (telecare) technologies work.
2. Of the patients in our survey, 42.3 per cent felt this action was difficult.
3. For a reflection on the naturalization of the fixed-line telephone, see Meyrowitz, 1985, p. 109.
4. Hartis. 'De Holterfoon. Handleiding voor de patient', p. 5 and 6.
5. Surveys 41 and 60; interviews 5, 6, 8, 9, 10, 11.
6. See Cooper, 2002, p. 24, who introduced the term 'indiscreet technologies' to refer to the capacity of the mobile phone to blur boundaries between discrete domains such as public and private and remote and distant.

7. Surveys 6, 15, 26, 27, 37, 47, 55, 68; interviews 2, 6, 10.
8. Replacing sound by light totally is, however, not an option. Sound signals are a prerequisite for the physician at the telemedical centre to be able to detect failures in sending ECGs by phone. Obviously, the designer has prioritized the physician as user over the patient as user. Another potential solution is that the sound be switched off during the recording, only leaving the beeps as signals for feedback on the other functions. Although the recorder provides this option, patients are not informed about this because it will make the recording too difficult: patients need the sound to confirm that they have activated the recorder correctly (Observation telemedical centre, January 19, 2005). The problem with the sensitive record button could have been solved by placing the button more deeply into the jacket of the recorder. These options to change the design were, however, not realized. The responsibility to solve these problems in use was thus delegated to the patients.
9. Surveys 6, 32, 37, 47, 55, 59.
10. Surveys 6, 8, 10, 41, 60, interviews 5, 6, 8, 9, 10, 11.
11. In the Netherlands, Home Care organizations are part of the regular healthcare system. They deliver services, including people and devices, to assist people to cope with disease and handicaps in their homes.
12. Although it would be worthwhile also to follow the assistants of physicians, I restricted the analysis to the work of home-care nurses at one Home Care organization in The Hague, a city centrally located in the Netherlands, that was the first Home Care organization enrolled by the Dutch distribution firm of ambulatory ECG-recorders to give instructions to patients.
13. Since spring 2005, the staff of telemedical centre have been available only during office hours (8 a.m.–8 p.m.) When patients call at night or on the weekends, their calls are transferred to a medical emergency call centre.
14. I use the male gender here because this observation concerned a male physician.
15. Of the patients in our survey, 34 per cent mentioned that they had hesitated to call the telecare centre because they were anxious to send an ECG that did not show any problem or did not want to disturb the physician at night.
16. I thank Adele Clarke for introducing this term.

Chapter 8

1. See Tweed, 2010 for a more detailed discussion of this phenomenological approach to spaces.
2. Interestingly, there is also another category of non-users involved in this story. Patients who participated in the clinical trial were allowed to use the telecare devices only for a limited period. After one year they had to hand in the devices as prescribed by the requirements of the clinical trial for this telemonitoring system. This situation exemplifies a situation in which users can become non-users again, not because they stop using the technology voluntarily, but because of loss of access. Patients who used the telemonitoring system thus became 'expelled' users, to use Wyatt's term for this category of non-users (Wyatt et al., 2002).

3. See Brown and Webster, 2004 for an exemplary study adopting this approach.
4. To guarantee that only patients and not visitors or family members could watch the graphs, the system could only be accessed by a password (Interview Sorgdrager, 2006).
5. Telenurses told us that they were inclined to answer any questions patients asked by phone but that they were instructed not to spend too much time on these calls. In case of frequent calls they had to tell the patient to keep it short or to go to their own physician (Interview Sorgdrager and Borst, 2006).
6. This finding confirms the study of Henwood and Wyatt on gendered patters in the use of Internet for seeking health information and making health-related decisions. Although the Internet, by making healthcare information accessible to women and men, has the potential to challenge the traditional gendered division of care work in which women bear the responsibility of health of family members, their research showed how these traditional gendered practices remained resistant to change (Henwood and Wyatt, 2009, p. 33).

Conclusions

1. See MobiHealth Project. European Commission. Information Society Technologies Program 2001–6 (www.mobihealth.org).
2. See Willems, 2006 for a similar conclusion about high-tech home-care technologies.
3. See Schermer, 2008 for an analysis of this debate.
4. See Pols et al., 2008 and Mort et al., 2008 for a similar argument about telecare technologies for elderly people.

Bibliography

Interviews

Germany

Albani, Marco. Supervisor at the Vitaphone Service Center in Chemnitz, 26 January 2005.

Gahlert, Cindy. Telenurse at the Vitaphone Service Center in Chemnitz, 26 January 2005.

Murin, Matthias. Director of Vitaphone Service Center in Chemnitz, 27 January 2005.

Quinger, Matthias. Works manager and co-founder of Vitaphone Germany, Mannheim, 7 December 2004 and 26 January 2005.

Sack, Stefan. Cardiologist at the Medical School of the University Hospital in Essen, 6 December 2004.

Wittig, Dieter. Telephysician at the Vitaphone Service Center in Chemnitz, 26 and 27 January 2005.

The Netherlands

Balk, Aggie. Cardiologist at the Erasmus Medical Centre in Rotterdam, 19 December 2005 and November 2007.

Beurs, Marielle de. Heart-failure nurse at the Onze Lieve Vrouwe Hospital (OLV) in Amsterdam, 18 December 2008.

Borst, Trix. Telephysician at the Achmea Medical Service Center, Zwolle, 28 March 2006.

Burgh, Pieter van der. Cardiologist at the Medical Spectrum Twente (MST) Hospital in Enschede, 21 August 2007.

Boutkan, Pieter. Project leader at Achmea Health in Amsterdam, 31 January 2006.

Dam, Claudia van. District nurse at the Home Care Centre in The Hague, 22 June 2004.

Helm, Mathilde. Research coordinator at Achmea Health in Amsterdam, 31 January 2006.

Glazenburg, Hanneke. Heart-failure nurse at the MST hospital in Enschede, 31 October 2006 and 30 May 2007.

Grooters, Judith. Heart-failure nurse at the MST hospital in Enschede, 12 October 2006.

Harthoorn, Sandra. District nurse at the Home Care Centre in The Hague, 22 June 2004.

Helm, Mathilde van der. Project leader of the heart-failure telemonitoring project at the health insurance company Achmea in Amsterdam, 31 January 2006.

Hollander, Tony den. Physician, Monnickendam, 22 June 2004.

Holwerda, Leo. Director Hartis B. V. Amsterdam, 4 May 2004.

Jurgens, Eric. Telephysician at the Hartis Telemedical Centre in Amsterdam, 4 May 2004 and 25 January 2005.

Kievit, Cora. Heart-failure nurse at the District hospital in Dirksland, 24 October 2007.
Leenders, C. M. Cardiologist at the hospital Havenziekenhuis in Rotterdam, 31 October 2007.
Leussen, Erwin van. Business manager, Achmea Health, Noordwijk 5 September 2007.
Margreet Woudenberg. Nurse practitioner at the Home Care Centre in The Hague, 3 September 2004.
Roukema, Janneke. Heart-failure nurse at the MST hospital in Enschede, 12 October 2006.
Schroeder, Jutta. Cardiologist at the OLV Hospital in Amsterdam, 18 December 2008.
Sorgdrager, Judith. Telenurse at the Achmea Medical Service Center, Zwolle, 28 March 2006.
Tongeren, Chris van. Regional manager at the Home Care Centre in The Hague, 22 June 2004.
Wal, Anita van der. Team leader at the Achmea Medical Service Center, Zwolle, 28 March 2006.
Weijde, Jelle van der. Manager Medical IT Benelux at Philips in Eindhoven, 29 May 2006.

Published sources

Abbott, A. 1988. *The System of Professions: An Essay on the Division of Expert Labor* (Chicago: University of Chicago Press).
Abraham, J., and Davis, C. 2007. "Deficits, expectations and paradigms in British and American drug safety assessment: opening the black box of regulatory science." *Science, Technology & Human Values* 32, nr. 4:399–343.
Achmea 2005. 'Philips en Achmea starten nieuw zorg-op-afstandsysteem.' (Achmea website June 9: 6).
Achmea Zorg Services 2006. 'Opleiding en training', *Project telemonitoring van patienten met chronisch hartfalen.*
Achmea and Philips. Press Information, 2005 (June 8).
Akrich, M. 1992. 'The De-scription of Technical Objects', in *Shaping Technology-Building Society: Studies in Sociotechnical Change*, eds W. Bijker and J. Law (Cambridge, MA, and London: MIT Press), p. 6, 205–44.
Akrich, M. and Latour, B. 1992. 'A summary of a Convenient Vocabulary for the Semiotics of Human and Nonhuman Assemblies', in *Shaping Technology/ Building Society: Studies in Sociotechnical Change*, eds W. E. Bijker and J. Law (Cambridge, MA, London, England: MIT Press).
Altenstetter, C. 2003. 'EU and Member State Medical Devices Regulation', *International Journal of Technology Assessment in Healthcare*, 19, no. 1: 228–48.
Andrews, G. J. 2002. 'Towards a More Place-sensitive Nursing Research: An Invitation to Medical and Health Geography', *Nursing Inquiry*, 9, no. 4: 221–38.
Andrews, G. J. 2003. 'Locating a Geography of Nursing: Space, Place and the Progress of Geographical Thought', *Nursing Philosophy*, 4: 231–48.
Angus, J., Kontos, P., Dyck, I., McKeever, P. and Poland, B. 2005. 'The Personal Significance of Home: Habitus and the Experience of Receiving Long-term Home Care', *Sociology of Health & Illness*, 27, no. 2: 161–87.

Annandale, E. and Kuhlmann, E. 2010. *The Palgrave Handbook of Gender and Healthcare* (Houndmills, Basingstoke, Hampshire: Palgrave Macmillan).

Anonymous 2002. *Telefoon Advies Systeem (TAS)*.

Anonymous 2003. 'Computer vervangt cardioloog', *ICT Zorg Nieuwsbrief,* (13 November), 1.

Anonymous 2004. *Beroepsdeelprofiel Hartfalenverpleegkundige: Algemene Vereniging Verpleegkundigen en verzorgenden* (Utrecht: Nederlandse Vereniging Hart-en Vaat Verpleegkundigen).

Anonymous 2005. 'Zorgverzekeraar stopt met huisartsenlijn', *Volkskrant* (January).

Anonymous 2008. 'Quality is Measurable', *Vitaphone Newsletter Telemedicine Today*, 3: 1.

Armstrong, P., Armstrong, H. and Laxer, K. 2007. 'Doubtful Data: Why Paradigms Matter in Counting the Health-care Labour Force', in *Work in Tumultuous Times: Critical Perspectives*, eds V. Shalla and W. Clement (Montreal and Kingston: McGill-Queens University Press), 326–48.

Armstrong, P., Armstrong, H. and Messing, K. 2009. 'Gendering Work? Women and Technologies in Health Care', in *Gender, Health and Information Technology in Context*, eds E. Balka, E. Green and F. Henwood (Houndsmill, Basingstoke, Hampshire: Palgrave Macmillan) 122–38.

Arras, J. D. and Neveloff Dubler, L. B. 1995. 'Introduction: Ethical and Social Implications of High-tech Home Care', in *Bringing the Hospital Home: Ethical and Social Implications of High-Tech Home Care*, eds J. D. Arras, W. H. Porterfield and L. O. Porterfield (Baltimore: The Johns Hopkins University Press), 1–31.

Balk, A. H. M. M., Leenders, C. M., Davidse, W. and Westerteicher, C. 2007. 'Personalised Tele-guidance of Heart Failure Patients: Effects of the MOTIVA Interactive Healthcare Platform on Hospital Admissions, Quality of Life, Knowledge of Disease and Self-care. A Pilot Study. Conference Heart Failure 2007 Organised by the Heart Failure Association of the European Society of Cardiology.' Poster Display III. Heart failure clinics.

Balka, E. Green, E. and Henwood, F. ed. 2009. *Gender, Health and Information Technology in Context* (Houndsmill, Basingstoke, Hampshire: Palgrave Macmillan).

Bauer, J. C. and Ringel, M. A. 1999. *Telemedicine and the Reinvention of Healthcare* (New York: McGraw-Hill).

Berg, M. 1997. 'Problems and Promises of the Protocol', *Social Science & Medicine*, 44: 1081–8.

Berg, M. and Mol, A. ed. 1998. *Difference in Medicine, Unravelling Practices, Techniques, and Bodies* (Durham and London: Duke University Press).

Bijker, W. E. 2007. 'American and Dutch Coastal Engineering', *Social Studies of Science*, 37, no. 1: 143–53.

Bjorn, P. and Balka, E. 2007. 'Health Care Categories Have Politics too: Unpacking the Managerial Agenda of Electronic Triage Systems', in *Proceedings of the 10th European Conference of Computer-Supported Cooperative Work*, eds L. Bannon, I. Wager, C. Gutwin, R. Harper and K. Schmidt (ECSCW Conference, Limerick, Ireland) 24–8 September 2007: 371–90.

Blume, S. 1992. *Insight and Industry: On the Dynamics of Technological Change in Medicine* (Cambridge: MIT Press).

Borup, M., Brown, N., Konrad, K. and Lente, H. 2006. 'The Sociology of Expectations in Science and Technology', *Technology Analysis & Strategic Management*, 18, no. 3/4, 2006: 286–98.

Bowker, G. C. and Star, S. L. 1999. *Sorting Things Out: Classification and Its Consequences* (Cambridge: MIT Press).

Brown, N. and Webster, A. 2004. *New Medical Technologies and Society: Reordering Life* (Cambridge and Maldan: Polity Press).

Callon, M. 1985. 'Some Elements of a Sociology of Translation: Domestication of Scallops and the Fishermen of St Brieu Bay', in *Power, Action, and Belief: Sociological Review Monograph*, ed. J. Law (London: Routledge and Kegan Paul).

Cairncross, F. 1997. *The Death of Distance: How the Communications Revolution Will Change our Lives* (Harvard Business School Press).

Cartier, C. 2003. 'From Home to Hospital and Back Again: Economic Restructuring, End of Life, and the Gendered Problems of Place-switching Services', *Social Science and Medicine*, 56: 2289–301.

Cartwright, L. 2000. 'Reach Out and Heal Someone: Telemedicine and the Globalisation of Healthcare', *Health*, 4, no. 3: 347–77.

Castells, M. 2000. *The Rise of the Network Society*, 2nd edn (Malden, MA: Blackwell).

Chetney, R. 2003. 'The Cardiac Connection Program', *Home Healthcare Nurse*, 21, no. 10: 680–6.

Clarke, A. E. and Montini, T. 1993. 'The Many Faces of RU486: Tales of Situated Knowledges and Technological Contestations', *Science, Technology and Human Values*, 18, no. 1: 42–78.

Clarke, A. 1998. *Disciplining Reproduction: Modernity, American Life and The Problem of Sex* (Chicago: Chicago University Press).

Clarke, A. E., Shim, J. K., Mamo, L., Fosket, J. R. and Fishman, J. R. 2003. 'Biomedicalization: Technoscientific Transformations of Health, Illness, and US Biomedicine', *American Sociological Review*, 68, no. 2: 161–94.

Clarke, A. E., Shim, J. K., Mamo, L., Fosket, J. R. and Fishman, J. R. 2010. 'Biomedicalization: A Theoretical and Substantive Introduction', in *Biomedicalization: Technoscience, Health, and Illness in the US*, eds A. E. Clarke, L. Mamo, J. R. Fosket, J. R. Fishman and J. K. Shim (Durham and London: Duke University Press).

Clausen, J. A. 2008. 'Producing Authoritative Knowledge: A Post-phenomenological Analysis of How Technologies Used for Fetal Surveillance Mediate Perception, Actions and Understanding of Child Birth', paper presented at the 4S-EASST conference, Rotterdam, August 2008.

Cleland, G. F., Louis, A. A., Rigby, A. S., Janssens, U. and Balk, H. M. M. 2005. 'Noninvasive Home Telemonitoring for Patients with Heart Failure at High Risk of Recurrent Admission and Death: The Trans-European Network-Home-Care Management System (TEN-HMS) Study', *Journal of the American College of Cardiology*, 45, no. 10: 1654–64.

Cooper, G. 2002. 'The Mutable Mobile: Social Theory in the Wireless World', in *Wireless World: Social and Interactional Aspects of the Mobile Age*, eds B. Brown, G. Green and R. Harper (London: Springer-verlag), 19–31.

Cowan, R. S. 1983. *More Work for Mother: The Ironies of Household Technology from the Open Hearth to the Microwave* (New York: Basic Books).

Crane, D. 1967. 'The Gatekeepers of Science: Some Factors Affecting the Selection of Articles in Scientific Journals', *American Sociologist*, 2: 195–201.

Currell, R., Urquhart, C. and Wainright, P. 2000. *Telemedicine Versus Face to Face Patient Care: Effects on Professional Practice and Healthcare Outcomes* (Chichester: John Wiley & Sons, The Cochrane Library).

DiMarco, J. P. and Philbrick, J. T. 1990. 'Use of Ambulatory Electrocardiographic (Holter) Monitoring', *Annals of Internal Medicine*, 113: 53–68.

Douglas, M. 1991. 'The Idea of Home: A Kind of Space', *Social Research*, 58, 1: 287–307.

Doyal, L. 2001. 'Sex, Gender and Health: The Need for a New Approach', *British Medical Journal*, 323, 1061–3.

Dubbeld, L. 2005. 'Privacy and Security Issues in Telemonitoring of Cardiac Patients', in *Computer Ethics: Philosophical Enquiry: Ethics of New Information Technology*, eds P. Brey, F. Grodzinsky, and L. Introna (Enschede: Universiteit Twente), 165–80.

Dubbeld, L. 2005. 'Protecting Personal Data in Camera Surveillance Practices', *Surveillance & Society*, 2: 546–63.

Edwards, B. 1994. 'Telephone Triage: How Experienced Nurses Reach Decisions', *Journal of Advanced Clinical Nursing*, 19: 717–24.

European Commission 2007. Communication on Telemedicine for the Benefits of Patients, Healthcare Systems and Society (Brussels).

Finch, T., May, C., Mort, M. and Mair, F. 2006. 'Telemedicine, Telecare, and the Future Patient: Innovation, Risk and Governance', in *New Technologies in Health Care: Challenge, Change and Innovation*, ed. A. Webster (Houndmills, Basingstoke, Hampshire: Palgrave Macmillan), 84–96.

Fischer, C. S. 1992. *America Calling: A Social History of the Telephone to 1940* (Berkeley, CA: University of California Press).

Foucault, M. 1973. *The Birth of the Clinic* (London: Routledge).

Foucault, M. 1988. 'Technologies of Self', in *Technologies of Self: A Seminar with Michel Foucault*, eds L. H. Martin, H. Gutman and P. H. Hutton (London: Tavistock Publications), 16–49.

Franklin, S. and Ragone, H. 1998. *Reproducing Reproduction: Kinship, Power, and Technological Innovation* (Philadelphia, Pennsylvania: University of Pennsylvania Press).

Freidson, E. 1975. *Doctoring Together: A Study of Professional Social Control* (New York: Elsevier).

Friedewald and Da Costa, 2003. 'Science and Technology Roadmapping: Ambient Intelligence in Everyday Life', in *Ageing, Technology and Home Care: New Actors, New Responsibilities*, eds M. Mort, C. Milligan, C. Roberts and I. Moser (Paris: Presses de l' Ecole des Mines) 2008.

Gasser, L. 1986. 'The Integration of Computing and Routine Work', *ACM Transactions on Office Information Systems*, 4: 257–70.

Giddens, A. 1991. *Modernity and Self-Identity: Self and Society in the Late Modern Age* (Cambridge: Polity Press).

Gieryn, T. F. 1983. 'Boundary-Work and the Demarcation of Science from Non-Science: Strains and Interests in Professional Ideologies of Scientists', *American Sociological Review*, 48: 781–95.

Gieryn, G. (1998) 'Biotechnology's Private Parts (and Some Public Ones)', in *Private Science: Biotechnology and the Rise of the Molecular Sciences*, ed. A. Thackray (Philadelphia: University of Pennsylvania Press), 219–53.

Gieryn, T. F. 2006. 'City as Truth-Spot: Laboratories and Field-Sites in Urban Studies', Social Studies of Science, 36, 1: 5–38.

Goffman, E. 1959. *The Presentation of the Self in Everyday Life* (New York: Doubleday).

Grinsven, L. van 2005. *Update 2 – Philips, Achmea Start TV Home Medical Care Trial*, Reuters News (June 8).

Halffman, W. 2003. *Boundaries of Regulatory Science: Eco/Toxicology and Aquatic Hazards of Chemicals in the US, England, and The Netherlands, 1970–1995* (Boechout: Albatros).

Hanlon, G., Strangleman, T., Goode, J., Luff, D., O'Cathain, A. and Greatbatch, D. 2005. 'Knowledge, Technology and Nursing: The Case of NHS Direct', *Human Relation*, 58, no. 2, 147–71.

Haraway, D. 1991. *Simians, Cyborgs, and Women: The Reinvention of Nature* (London: Free Association Books and New York: Routledge).

Hardt, M. 1999. 'Affective Labour', *Boundary*, 26, no. 2: 89–100.

Harvey, D. 1990. *The Condition of Postmodernity: An Enquiry into the Origins of Cultural Change* (Cambridge, MA: Blackwell).

Heaton, J., Noyes, J., Sloper, P. and Shah, R. 2005. 'Families Experiences of Caring for Technology-dependent Children: A Temporal Perspective', *Health and Social Care in the Community*, 13, no. 2: 22–40.

Henke, C. R. and T. F. Gieryn 2008. 'Sites of Scientific Practice: The Enduring Importance of Place', in *Handbook of Science and Technology Studies*, eds E. J. Hacket, O. Amsterdamska, M. Lynch and J. Wajcman (Massachusetts: MIT Press), 1–29.

Henwood, F., Kennedy, H. and N. Miller (eds) 2001. *Cyborg Lives? Women's Technobiographies* (Raw Nerve Books).

Henwood, F., Wyatt, S., Hart, A. and Smith, J. 2003. '"Ignorance is Bliss Sometimes": Constraints on the Emergence of the "Informed Patient" in the Changing Landscapes of Health Information', *Sociology of Health & Illness*, 25, no. 6: 589–607.

Henwood, F. and Wyatt S. 2009. 'All Change? Gender, Health and the Internet', in *Informing Gender? Health and Information Technologies in Context*, eds E. Balka, E. Green and F. Henwood (Houndmills: Palgrave Macmillan), 17–33.

Houwaart, E. S. 2001. 'Van Medisch instrument naar medisch-technologisch system', in *Techniek in Nederland in de twintigste eeuw*, Deel IV, J. W. Schot e. a. (red.). (Zutphen: Walburg Pers). 163–79.

Illich, I. 1981. *Shadow Work* (Boston: Marion Boyars).

Inspectie Gezondheidszorg 2003. *Staat van de gezondheidszorg. Deelrapport onderzoek naar ketenzorg bij chronisch hartfalen* (Den Haag: Inspectie Gezondheidszorg).

Irwin, A. and Michael, M. 2003. *Science, Social Theory and Public Knowledge* (Maidenhead: Open University Press).

Johnson Pettinari, C. J. and Jessopp, L. 2001. 'Issues and Innovations in Nursing Practice: "Your Ears Become Your Eyes": Managing the Absence of Visibility in NHS Direct', *Journal of Advanced Nursing*, 36, no. 5: 668–75.

Johnson-Mekota, J. L., Maas, M., Buresh, K. A., Gardner, S. E., Frantz, R. A., Pringle Specht, J. K., Wakefield, B. and Flanagan, J. 2001. 'A Nursing Application of Telecommunications: Measurement of Satisfaction for Patients and Providers', *Journal of Gerontological Nursing*, 27: 28–33.

Johnston Roberts, K. 1999. 'Patient Empowerment in the United States: A Critical Commentary', *Health Expectation*, 2: 82–92.

Katz, J. E. and Aspden, P. 1998. 'Internet Dropouts in the USA, The Invisible Group', *Telecommunications Policy*, 22, no. 4/5: 327–39.

Kendall, L. 2001. *The Future Patient* (London: Institute of Public Policy Research).

Kennedy, H. 2003. 'Technobiography: Researching Lives, Online and Off', *Biography*, vol. 26.

Kirejczyk, M. 2000. 'Enculturation Through Script Selection: Political Discourse and Practice of In Vitro Fertilization in The Netherlands', in *Bodies of Technology: Women's Involvement with Reproductive Medicine*, eds A. R. Saetnan, N. Oudshoorn and M. Kirejczyk (Columbus: Ohio University Press), 183–207.

Kline, R. 2000. *Consumers in the Country: Technology and Social Change in Rural America* (Baltimore and London: Johns Hopkins University Press).

Kline, R. 2003. 'Resisting Consumer Technology in Rural America: The Telephone and Electrification', in *How Users Matter: The Co-construction of Users and Technology*, eds N. Oudshoorn, and T. J. Pinch (Massachusetts and London: MIT Press), 51–69.

Kline, R. and Pinch, T. 1996. 'Users as Agents of Technological Change: The Social Construction of the Automobile in the Rural United States', *Technology and Culture*, 37, no. 4: 763–95.

Kolko, J. 2000. 'The Death of Cities? The Death of Distance? Evidence from the Geography of Commercial Internet Usage', in *The Internet Upheaval: Raising Questions, Seeking Answers in Communications Policy*, eds J. Vogelsang and B. M. Compaine (Cambridge, MA, London, England: The MIT Press).

Konrad, K. 2006. 'The Social Dynamics of Expectations: The Interaction of Collective and Actor-Specific Expectations on Electronic Commerce and Interactive Television', *Technology Analysis & Strategic Management*, 18, no. 3/4: 429–44.

Langstrup Nielsen, H. 2003. 'Self-monitoring: IT and the Construction of the Competent Patient', Papers in Organization, no. 50, Copenhagen Business School.

Larson, Magali Sarfatti 1979. 'Professionalism: Rise and Fall', *Journal of Health Services*, 9, no. 4: 607–27.

Latour, B. 1987. *Science in Action* (Cambridge: Harvard University Press).

Latour, B. 1988. 'Mixing Humans and Nonhumans Together: The Sociology of a Door-closer', *Social Problems*, 35, no. 3: 298–310.

Latour, B. 1989. 'Clothing the Naked Truth', in *Dismantling Truth: Reality in the Post-Modern World*, eds H. Lawson and L. Appignanesi (Weidenfeld & Nicholson), 101–28.

Latour, B. 1990. 'The Force and Reason of Experiment', in *Experimental Inquiries, Historical, Philosophical and Social Studies of Experimentation in Science*, ed. Homer Le Grand (Dordrecht: Kluwer Academic Publishers), 48–79.

Latour, B. 2005. *Reassembling the Social* (Oxford University Press).

Law, J. 1999. 'After ANT: Complexity, Naming and Topology', in *Actor Network Theory and After*, eds J. Law and J. Hassards (Oxford: Blackwell Publishers).

Law, J. 2008. 'Actor-Network Theory and Material Semiotics', in *The New Blackwell Companion to Social Theory 3rd Edn*, ed. B. S. Turner (Blackwell), pp. 141–58.

Lehoux, P., Sicotte, C., Denis, J.-L., Berg, M., Lacroix, A. 2002. "The theory of use behind telemedicine: how compatible with physicians' clinical routines?" *Social Science & Medicine*, 54: 889–904.

Lehoux, P. 2006. *The Problem of Health Technology: Policy Implications for Modern Health Care Systems* (New York and London: Routledge, Taylor & Francis).

Lehoux, P., Saint-Arnaud, J. and Richard, L. 2004. 'The Use of Technology at Home: What Patient Manuals Say and Sell vs What Patients Face and Fear', *Sociology of Health & Illness*, 5: 617–44.

Lehrer, K. 1990. *Theory of Knowledge* (London: Routledge).

Lente, H. and Rip, A. 1998. 'Expectations in Technological Developments: An Example of Prospective Structures to be Filled in by Agency', in *Getting New Technologies Together: Studies in Making Sociotechnical Order*, eds C. D. Disco and B. van der Meulen (Berlin and New York: Walter de Gruyter), 203–29.

Livingstone, D. N. 2003. *Putting Science in Its Place: Geographies of Scientific Knowledge* (Chicago: University of Chicago Press).

Lopez, D. 2010. 'Exploring the Affordances of Telecare-related Technologies in the Home', in *New Technologies and Emerging Spaces of Care*, eds M. Schillmeijer and M. Domenech (Surrey and Burlington: Ashgate), 39–57.

Maathuis, I. 2005. Transcript Meeting Representatives Vitaphone and Vodaphone.

Mackay, H., Crane, C., Beynon-Davies, P. and Tudhope, D. 2000. 'Reconfiguring the User: Using Rapid Application Development', *Social Studies of Science*, 30, no. 5: 737–59.

Mair, F. S., Hibbert, D., May, C. R., Angus, R., Finch, T., Boland, A., OConnor, J., Haycox, A., Roberts, C., and Capewell, S. 2004. 'Problems with Implementation: The Story of a Home Telecare Trial', in *Understanding Health Communication Technologies*, eds P. Whitten and D. Cook (San Francisco: John Wiley & Sons), 3–10.

Malone, R. E. 2003. 'Distal Nursing', *Social Science & Medicine*, 56: 2317–26.

Maltha, S., Bongers, F., Schuurman K., Vandeberg R., Vermaas, K. and Van Wijngaert, L. 2003. *Breedband en de gebruiker* (Utrecht: Dialogic).

Marvin, C. 1988. *When Old Technologies Were New: Thinking about Electric Communication in the Late Nineteenth Century* (New York: Oxford University Press).

Mattke, S. 'Health and Well-being in the Home: Study Overview', Paper presented at the International Congress on Telehealth and Telecare, London, 1–3 March 2011.

May, C. R., Mort, M. Finch, T. and Mair, F. S. 2004. 'The Anatomy of Failure? Teledermatology in an English city', in *Understanding Health Communication Technologies*, eds P. Whitten, and D. Cook (San Francisco: John Wiley & Sons), 80–7.

May, C., Finch, T., Mair, F. and Mort, M. 2005. 'Towards a Wireless Patient: Chronic Illness, Scarce Care and Technological Innovation in the United Kingdom', *Social Science & Medicine*, 61: 1485–94.

May, C., Mort, M., Mair, F. and Finch, T. 2007. 'Telemedicine and the "Future Patient"? Risk, Governance and Innovation', *Innovative Health Technologies*. (http://www.york.ac.uk/res/iht/projects/l218252067/MayFinalRptSummary Refs.pdf: November 27).

McDonald, I. G., Daly, J., Jelinek, V. M., Panetta, F., Gutman, J. M. 1996. 'Opening Pandora's Box: The Unpredictability of Reassurance, by a Normal Test Result', *British Medical Journal*, 313: 329–32.

McDowell, L. 1999. Gender, Identity and Place: Understanding Feminist Geographies (University of Minnesota Press).

McKeever, P. 2001. 'Home Care in Canada: Housing Matters', *Canadian Journal of Nursing Research*, 33, no. 2: 3–4.

Merleau-Ponty, M. 1962 *The Phenomenology of Perception* (Routledge and Kegan Paul Ltd.)

Meyrowitz, J. 1985. *No Sense of Place: The Impact of Electronic Media on Social Behaviour* (Oxford: Oxford University Press).

Michael, M. 1996. 'Technologies and Tantrums: Hybrids out of Control in the Case of Road Rage', Paper presented at the 'Signatures of Knowledge Societies'. Joint 4S/EASST conference at the University of Bielefeld, Germany, October 10–13.

Milligan, C. 2001. *Geographies of Care: Space, Place and the Voluntary Sector* (Aldershot, Burlington USA, Singapore, and Sydney: Ashgate).

Milligan, C., Atkinson, S., Skinner, M. and Wiles, J. 2007. *Geographies of Care – A Critical Commentary* (New Zealander Geographer).

Milligan, C. 2009. *There's No Place Like Home: Place and Care in an Ageing Society* (Aldershot, Burlington USA, Singapore, and Sydney: Ashgate).

Milligan, M., Mort, M. and C. Roberts, 2010. 'Cracks in the Door? Technology and the Shifting Topology of Care', in *New Technologies and Emerging Spaces of Care*, eds M. Schillmeijer and M. Domenech (Surrey and Burlington: Ashgate), 19–39.

Mol, A. 2002. *The Body Multiple: Ontology in Medical Practice* (Durham and London: Duke University Press).

Mol, A. 2008. *The Logic of Care* (London: Routledge).

Mol, A., Moser, I., and Polis, J. 2010 (eds) *Care in Practice. On Tinkering in Clinics, Homes and Farms* (Bielefeld: Transcript Verlag).

Montfoort, A. P. W. P. and Helm, M. H. J. van der. 2006. 'Telemonitoring of Patients with Chronic Heart Failure', *Disease Management & Health Outcomes*, 14, no. 1: 33–5.

Moore, M. 1999, 'The Evolution of Telemedicine', *Future Generations Computer Systems*, 15: 245–54.

Mort, M., May, C. R. and Williams, T. 2003. 'Remote Doctors and Absent Patients: Acting at a Distance in Telemedicine?', *Science, Technology, & Human Values*, 28, no. 2: 274–95.

Mort, M., May, C., Williams, T. and Mair, F. 2004. 'From Convergence to Confidence: Science, Technology and Politics in Telemedicine', in *Governing Medicine: Theory and Practice*, eds A. Gray and S. Harrison (Buckingham: Open Unversity Press).

Mort, M., Finch, T. and C. May 2009. 'Making and Unmaking Telepatients: Identity and Governance in New Health Technologies', *Science, Technology and Human Values*, 34, no. 1: 9–33.

Mort, M., Milligan, C., Roberts, C. and Moser, I. 2008. *Ageing, Technology and Home Care: New Actors, New Responsibilities* (Paris: Presses de l'Ecole des Mines. Collection Science Sociales).

Mort, M., Roberts, C. and C. Milligan (eds) 2009. 'Ageing, Technology and the Home: A Critical Project', *ALTER, European Journal of Disability*, 3, 85–9.

Moser, I. 2008. 'Mediating Loving Care or Vital Signs? The Sociality of Care Technologies', in *Ageing, Technology and Home care: New Actors and New Responsibilities*, eds M. Mort, C. Milligan, C. Roberts and I. Moser (Paris: Presses de l' Ecole des Mines. Collection Science Sociales), 73–4.

Murin, M. 2005. Presentation Meeting Vitaphone and Vodaphone, 2005.

Nettleton, S. 2004. 'The Emergence of E-scaped Medicine', *Sociology*, 38, no. 4: 661–80.

Nettleton, S. 2006. *Sociology of Health and Illness* 2nd edn (Cambridge: Polity Press).

Norcliffe, G. 2009. 'G-COT: The Geographical Construction of Technology', *Science, Technology and Human Values*, 34, no. 4: 449–75.

Oudshoorn, N. and Pinch, T. ed. 2003. *How Users Matter The Co-Construction of Users and Technologies* (MIT Press).

Oudshoorn, N., Brouns, M. and van Oost, E. 2005. 'Diversity and Distributed Agency in the Design and Use of Medical Video-Communication Technologies', in *Inside the Politics of Technology*, ed. H. Harbers (Amsterdam University Press).

Oudshoorn, N. and Pinch, T. 2007. 'User-Technology Relationships: Some Recent Developments', in *The Handbook of Science and Technology Studies*, eds E. J. Hackett, O. Amsterdamska, M. Lynch and J. Wajcman (The MIT Press).

Philips. Press Information 2004. 'Philips to begin pilot study of TV-based solution to help patients manage their health from home.' (October 15).

Philips. Press Information 2005. 'US study shows chronic disease patients embrace Philips personalized TV-based interactive healthcare platform to manage disease from home.' (June 8).

Philips. 2005. 'Monitoring your heart condition via your cell phone? It's not out of the question.' (www.newscenter.philips.com – article – 14758. downloaded November 25).

Philips. Press Information 2006. 'Philips announces US commercial launch of Motiva – a TV-based platform for remote patient management.' (May 8).

Philips 2005. *Bringing It All Back Home*. Flyer.

Philips and Achmea 2005. 'Philips and Achmea to launch first European pilot study of TV-based system for patients to manage health at home.' Press information June 8 2005.

Pickstone, J. V. 2000. 'Production, Community and Consumption: The Political Economy of Twentieth Century Medicine.' in *Medicine in the Twentieth Century*, eds R. Cooter and J. Pickstone (Amsterdam: Harwood Academic).

Poland, B., Lehoux, P., Holmes, D. and G. Andrews 2005. 'How Place Matters: Unpacking Technology and Power in Health and Social Care', *Health and Social Care*, 13, no. 2: 170–80.

Pols, J. 2008. 'Wonderful Webcams: About Active and Invisible Technologies', in *Care at a Distance: A Normative Investigation into Telecare: The Paper*, eds J. Pols, M. Schermer, C. Ploem and D. Willems (Amsterdam: AMC Amsterdam).

Pols, J., Schermer, M. and Willems, D. 2008. *Telezorgvisie. Essay over ontwikkelingen en beloften van telezorg in de Nederlandse gezondheidszorg* (NWO, Erasmus Universiteit en AMC, Universiteit van Amsterdam).

Prout, A. 1996. 'Actor–Network Theory, Technology and Medical Sociology: An Illustrative Analysis of the Metered Dose Inhaler', *Sociology of Health & Illness*, 18, no. 2: 198–219.

Roberts, C. and Mort, M. 2009. 'Reshaping what Counts as Care: Older People, Work and New Technologies', *ALTER, European Journal of Disability*, 3, 138–58.

Rogers, E. M. 2003. *Diffusion of Innovation* Fifth Edn (New York: Free Press).

Rommes, E. 2002. *Gender Scripts and the Internet: The Design and Use of Amsterdam's Digital City*, Ph.D. Dissertation University of Twente (The Netherlands).

Rowles, G. D. 1993. 'Evolving Images of Place in Aging and Aging in Place', *Generations*, 17, 2: 51–65.

Royal Philips Electronics 2008. EU project aims to help heart patients through telemonitoring. *Hospital healthcare.com: The Online Resource for Senior Management in Hospitals across Europe.* www.hospitalhealthcare.com. (Downloaded March 3).

Saetnan, A. R., Oudshoorn, N. and M. Kirejczyk (eds) 2000. *Bodies of Technology: Women's Involvement with Reproductive Medicine* (Columbus: Ohio State University Press).

Santen, H. 2008. 'Zorgvuldig opereren', *NRC Handelsblad*, (July 19).

Schermer, M. 2008. 'Telecare: New Ethical Issues in Selfmanagement, Compliance and Patients' Duties', in *Care at a Distance: A Normative Investigation into Telecare: The Papers*, eds J. Pols, M. Schermer, C. Ploem, and D. Willems (Amsterdam: Amsterdam Medisch Centrum), 13–24.

Schillmeijer, M. and Domenech, M. 2010. 'New Technologies and Emerging Spaces – An Introduction', in *New Technologies and Emerging Spaces of Care*, eds M. Schillmeijer and M. Domenech (Surrey and Burlington: Ashgate), 1–19.

Schmidt, K. and Simone, C. 1996. 'Coordination Mechanisms: Towards a Conceptual Foundation of CSCW Systems Design', *Computer Supported Cooperative Work: The Journal of Collaborative Computing*, 5: 155–200.

SCP. 2005. *Sociaal en Cultureel Rapport 2004: Hoofdstuk 5 ICT en Samenleving* (Den Haag: Sociaal Cultureel Planbureau (SCP)).

Selwyn, N. 2003. 'Apart from Technology: Understanding People's Non-use of Information and Communication Technologies in Everyday Life', *Technology in Society*, 25: 99–116.

Silverstone, R., Hirsch, E. and Morley, D. 1992. 'Information and Communication Technologies and the Moral Economy of the Household', in *Consuming Technologies, Media and Information in Domestic Spaces*, eds R. Silverstone and E. Hirsch (London: Routledge).

Silverstone R., and Haddon, L. 1996. "Design and the domestication of information and communication technologies: Technical change and everyday life," in *Communication by Design. The Politics of Information and Communication Technologies*, R. Silverstone, and R. Mansell, eds. Oxford: Oxford University Press, 44–74.

Spelten, E. R. and Gubbels, J. W. 2003. 'Een medisch callcenter in de praktijk. Onderzoek naar effect en ervaring', *Huisarts&Wetenschap*, 26: 543–6.

Star, S. L. 1989. *Regions of the Mind: Brain Research and the Quest for Scientific Certainty* (Stanford, CA: Stanford University Press).

Star, S. L. 1991. 'Power, Technologies and the Phenomenology of Conventions: On Being Allergic to Onions', in *The Sociology of Monsters, Essays on Power, Technology and Domination*, ed. J. Law (London: Routledge), 26–56.

Star, S. L. 1999. 'The Ethnography of Infrastructure', *American Behavioral Scientist*, 43, no. 3, 377–91.

Star, S. L. and Strauss, A. 1999. 'Layers of Silence, Arenas of Voice: The Ecology of Visible and Invisible Work', *Computer Supported Work*, 8: 9–30.

Strauss, A. 1985. 'Work and the Division of Labor', *The Sociological Quarterly*, 26: 1–19.

Strauss, A. L., Fagerhaugh, S., Suczek, B. and Wiener, C. 1997. *Social Organization of Medical Work* (New Brunswick and London: Transaction Publishers).

Sturken, M., Thomas, D. and Ball-Rokeach, S. J. ed. 2004. *Technological Visions: The Hopes and Fears that Shape New Technologies* (Philadelphia, PA: Temple University Press).

Suchman, L. 2002. 'Practice Based Design of Information Systems: Notes from the Hyperdeveloped World', *The Information Society*, 18: 139–44.

Suchman, L. 1994. 'Do Categories Have Politics? The Language/Action Perspective Reconsidered', *Computer Supported Cooperative Work (CWCW): An International Journal*, 2: 177–90.

Timmermans, S. and Berg, M. 2003. 'The Practice of Medical Technology', *Sociology of Health & Illness*, 25: 97–114.

Townly, B. 2002. 'Managing Modernity', *Organization*, 9: 549–73.

Tuan, Y. -F. 2004. *Home in Patterned Ground: The Entanglements of Nature and Culture*, eds S. Harrison, S. Pile and N. Thrift (London: Reaktion Books), Website Hartis (www.hartis.nl), downloaded 13 April 2006, 164–5.

Tweed, C. 2010. 'Exploring the Affordances of Telecare-related Technologies in the Home', in *New Technologies and Emerging Spaces of Care*, eds M. Schillmeijer and M. Domenech (Surrey and Burlington: Ashgate), 57–77.

Vitaphone 2006. *eHealth can provide solutions*. Brochure downloaded from Vitaphone's website (May 31: 7).

Wahlberg, A., Cedersund, E. and Wredling, R. 2003. 'Telephone Nurses Experience of Problems with Telephone Advice in Sweden', *Journal of Clinical Nursing*, 12: 37–45.

Webster, A. J. 2002. 'Innovative Health Technologies and the Social: Redefining Health, Medicine and the Body', *Current Sociology* 50: 443–57.

Webster, A. ed. 2006. *New Technologies in Healthcare: Challenge, Change and Innovation* (Houndmills, Basingstoke, Hampshire: Palgrave Macmillan).

Webster, A. 2007. *Health, Technology & Society: A Sociological Critique* (Houndmills, Basingstoke, Hampshire: Palgrave Macmillan).

Willems, D. 1995. *Tools of Care: Explorations into the Semiotics of Medical Technology*, Ph.D.-dissertation University of Limburg, The Netherlands.

Willems, D. 2006. *'Moral Machinery: Medical High Tech in the Home'*, Paper presented at Lancaster University seminar series, Perspectives in Science, Technology & Medicine (May 4).

Willems, D. 2008. 'Homes as in: Home Care Technologies', in *Ageing, Technology and Home Care: New Actors and New Responsibilities*, eds M. Mort, C. Milligan, C. Roberts and I. Moser (Paris: Presses de l' Ecole des Mines. Collection Science Sociales), 62–3.

Willems, D. 2010. 'Varieties of Goodness in High-tech Home Care', in *Care in Practice: On Tinkering in Clinics, Homes and Farms*, eds A. Mol, I. Moser and J. Pols (Bielefeld: Transcript Verlag. Series MatteRealities/Verkorperungen. Perspectives from Empirical Science Studies, vol. 8), 257–77.

Wootton, R. 2000. 'The Development of Telemedicine', in *Taking Health Telematics into the 21st Century*, eds M. Rigby, Thick, B. (Abington: Radcliffe Medical Press), 17–25.

Wyatt, S. 2003. 'Non-users also Matter: The Co-construction of Users and Non-users of the Internet', in *How Users Matter: The Co-construction of Users and Technology*, eds N. Oudshoorn and T. J. Pinch (Massachusetts and London: MIT Press), 68–9.

Wyatt, S., Thomas, G. and Terranova, T. 2002. 'They Came, They Surfed, They Went Back to the Beach: Conceptualising Use and Non-use of the Internet', in *Virtual Society? Technology, Cyberbole, Reality*, ed. S. Woolgar (Oxford: Oxford University Press), 23–40.

Zhao. S. 2005. 'The Digital Self: Through the Looking Glass of Telecopresent Others', *Symbolic Interaction*, 28 no. 3: 387–405.

Zilveren Kruis/Achmea 2008. *Overzicht vergoedingen Beter Af Polis en Aanvullende Verzekeringen.*

Index

Index 241

as invisible labour 91–2
see also telenurses; telephysicians
telemedical centres 7–8, 12, 25, 42,
51–2, 73, 78–9, 125, 127, 139–41
bypassing of 84–6
Germany 92–7, 110–18
negative perceptions of 80–3
Netherlands 92, 94, 97–110,
132–5, 160
telemonitoring
heart attacks 47–55, 77–80
heart-rhythm disturbances 55–62
and telemedical centres 98
see also individual devices/systems
telemonitoring systems 107, 109,
113–17, 132
alternatives to 172, 181–5
clinical trials 125
telenurses 4, 12, 42, 96–7, 101–2,
105, 107–8, 110–13, 115, 134–8,
140
telephone-based services 8, 98–9,
101–2, 126
telephysicians 12, 106, 108–9, 111,
113–15, 117, 135–6
invisible labour of 160–5
temporal dimension 134–5, 139
Timmermans, S. 14
Townly, B. 104
traditional healthcare actors 41–2,
52, 54–5, 63, 70, 78, 92, 104–5,
117, 196
training 107, 116–17, 136
of patients 148–9, 158–9
triage advice system 98, 101–4,
107–9, 134, 138

trust 156, 162
Tuan, Y.-F. 169

UK 8, 15, 107, 118, 122, 172,
192–3
US 8, 15, 21, 29, 37–9, 41–2, 44, 51,
69, 71, 76, 85, 101, 172, 211
user-technology relations 10, 17, 19,
25, 27–8, 42–3, 98, 148–53, 171

visual cues 128–9, 136–8
Vitaphone 29, 47–55, 58, 62, 68,
71–4, 92–3, 95–7, 110, 112–13
vulnerability 151

Wahlberg, A. 8, 122, 126, 165
Wal, A. van der 96–7, 100, 102,
105–6, 135, 137
Webster, A. 6–7, 15, 20, 25–6, 63,
125, 146, 195
Weijde, J. van der 41, 78, 81
Willems, D. 6, 17, 24, 66, 153, 180,
187–8, 198–9
Wittig, D. 96, 115, 117
Wootton, R. 9
work-arounds 105–10, 116–17, 135,
192–3
work practice 99–101, 106–7,
111–18
polyclinics 127–9
telemedical centres 160–2
World Health Organization 13, 15,
202
Wyatt, S. 28, 171, 179

Zhao, S. 176

Printed in the United States
By Bookmasters